THE TONGUE
as a Gateway to
Voice, Resonance,
Style, and Intelligibility

THE TONGUE
as a Gateway to Voice, Resonance, Style, and Intelligibility

Angelika Nair, PhD

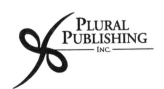

PLURAL
PUBLISHING
INC.

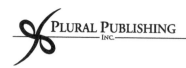

5521 Ruffin Road
San Diego, CA 92123

e-mail: information@pluralpublishing.com
Website: https://www.pluralpublishing.com

Typeset in 10.5/13 Minion Pro by Flanagan's Publishing Services, Inc.
Printed in the United States of America by Integrated Books International

Library of Congress Cataloging-in-Publication Data:
Names: Nair, Angelika, author.
Title: The tongue as a gateway to voice, resonance, style, and
    intelligibility / Angelika Nair.
Description: San Diego, CA : Plural Publishing, Inc., [2021] | Includes
    bibliographical references and index.
Identifiers: LCCN 2021002984 (print) | LCCN 2021002985 (ebook) | ISBN
    9781635503630 (paperback) | ISBN 1635503639 (paperback) | ISBN
    9781635503647 (ebook)
Subjects: MESH: Voice—physiology | Tongue—physiology | Speech—physiology
Classification: LCC QP306 (print) | LCC QP306 (ebook) | NLM WV 501 | DDC
    612.7/8—dc23
LC record available at https://lccn.loc.gov/2021002984
LC ebook record available at https://lccn.loc.gov/2021002985

Contents

Foreword

The human voice has been receiving increased attention from researchers, scholars, clinicians, and vocal pedagogues all over the world. Abstract rhetorical and metaphorical discourse has been replaced with detailed scientific information offered by colleagues from different academic backgrounds.

It is a pleasure to introduce to the voice audience this book by Angelika Nair, a thoughtful, intriguing, and fascinating text on the human voice. This book makes a unique contribution to the field in two major respects. First, Dr. Nair translates the complex nature of voice science into simple terms, practically applicable to anyone who wants to enhance his or her training, performance, teaching, or voice awareness. Second, she explores the voice as a whole, giving attention not only to phonation and the voice box itself, but also to whole vocal product as the result of a sophisticated transformation of the basic sound through the vocal tract. Tongue and mandible are not treated as components of the vocal tract but as important elements of interconnectedness with the entire voice box, which makes complete sense. The world of voice is predominantly based on vowels, the so-called "vowel centric world"; however, consonants have resonance, and this may interfere with the quality of the vocal output. Beautiful ultrasound images are offered to give insights on the inner process of singing and also to help improve speaking. Moreover, Dr. Nair shares with the reader her experience using biofeedback in the voice studio. Consonants and tongue are never going to be overlooked again.

This book has updated scientific information, but beyond that, it is a practical resource with exercises, step-by-step instructions, and graphics/illustrations that make it engaging and easy to follow, with immediate applications. Special attention has to be given to the illustrations, all made by the author. They are simple, precise, and attractive—a tough combination when showing anatomical landmarks and specific movements' details. The integration of drawings and ultrasound imaging is unique; I am sure that these figures are going to be used in classes, congresses, and courses all over the world. The whole text plus the exercises enable the reader to visualize the hidden nature of voice production, thus helping with the execution. For example, how to manipulate the tongue for maximum consonant resonance is clearly presented.

A final word should be said on the intense presence of Prof. Garyth Nair between the lines of this book. Those who had the privilege of meeting him surely remember quite well his intelligence, high expectations, and intense criticism of the obscurantism of some approaches to vocal pedagogy. The arrival of Dr. Angelika Nair in his life produced a strong combination of their talents, with immediate scientific and pedagogic results that were presented in conferences across the United States and abroad. She has not only maintained but also upgraded this legacy by challenging and motivating herself to write this book. I deeply recognize and appreciate her efforts, even if I can barely grasp the mix of emotions that must have been involved in this process.

I wish all colleagues a good reading of this book, with confidence that not only the knowledge it contains but also the passion for the human voice will be perceived throughout its chapters.

Mara Behlau, PhD
Director of Centro de Estudos
    da Voz–CEV, São Paulo, Brazil
Permanent Professor of the
    Graduate Program in Human
    Communicative Disorders at
    Universidade Federal de São
    Paulo—Escola Paulista de
    Medicina, São Paulo, Brazil

Preface

Life can be full of surprises. And I certainly had a lot of them in mine, including publishing this book. Writing a book is always a long endeavor, particularly if it is the first one. In this case it is both the first book I have written and a continuation of my mission to show that there is no dichotomy between voice science and voice pedagogy.

It all started with Garyth Nair's first book *Voice Tradition and Technology: A State-of-the-Art Studio* (Singular Publishing, 1999) in which he merged new knowledge into musical training by integrating computer-assisted, real-time analysis through spectrography. This was, as Sataloff wrote, "a milestone in the interdisciplinary evolution of vocal art and science."[1] A couple years later, his second book *The Craft of Singing* (Plural Publishing, 2007) came out in which he applied the current knowledge about voice function to the art of singing.

Now, this book continues in the same spirit, merging new knowledge—particularly about the tongue shapes and movements in resonant vocal production—into vocal training by integrating ultrasound as biofeedback.

How did I get from being a professional singer and experienced voice pedagogue to doing voice research? The journey started with both my curiosity to always know the how *and* why, the instinctual sense that there is more to singing (and teaching voice) than what I had learned in my studies. Listening to and watching the best of the best in the classical singing world, I observed a lot that I was not able to copy, let alone understand the physiology. So, I went on a personal mission and started researching, reading every book there is, attending workshops, and the like. But it was not until I looked for literature outside the German-speaking countries that a whole new world opened up to me: voice research. It was a steep learning curve working through the literature primarily written for, and by, scientists and clinicians. Trust me, I wished I would have already had the training to become a vocologist at the National Center for Voice and Speech (Salt Lake City, Utah) back then. But that did not yet exist. Anyway, eventually, I found Garyth Nair's first book and instantly felt as if he was writing from my own heart. Little did I know that this bibliographic love at first sight would literally become the love of my life.

Fast-forward, I not only found the love of my life, but also a man with whom I could share intellectually and professionally. So, I became Garyth's research partner, and together we continued his legacy of finding new insight into voice science and making it applicable to everyday teaching methods and voice use. In this spirit, we started to conduct groundbreaking research together, investigating the physiology of the low mandible maneuver (LMM; drop of the posterior mandible) and its ramification

---

[1]Garyth Nair, *Voice Tradition and Technology: A State-of-the-Art Studio* (San Diego, CA: Singular Publishing, 1999), ix.

for resonance production, as well as the rehabituation of tongue shapes required for all phonemes in high-ranking singers. In preparation for this research, we knew that we needed to use various imagery techniques. The collaboration with the Austrian Medical University of Graz was one major and generous puzzle piece. Our goal to have equipment that can be broken down for transportation to remote locations—singers' homes, studios, dressing rooms, and so forth—led us to ultrasound, and ultimately to Dr. Maureen Stone of the University of Maryland, who originally developed the technique of the acquisition of midsagittal (the midline slice) tongue profiles.

Dr. Stone generously invited us to come to her lab to introduce us to the ultrasound, and to explore its use for our purposes. I will never forget how ecstatic, fascinated, and astounded we were seeing our tongue in action during singing. It felt like Christmas, Easter, and every other feast and birthday wrapped in one. We just could not believe what we saw, experimented for hours, and recorded a protocol for further study. Before long, it became clear that this would be a major part in our research. So, for our LMM study we used magnetic resonance imaging, ultrasound, and spectrographic techniques and collected enough data to analyze for years. We even purchased our own portable ultrasound machine, knowing that we would continue using it for research and teaching. In June of 2013, with preliminary results, we presented as well as won first prize with our poster at the Voice Foundation's annual symposium in Philadelphia, Pennsylvania. Tragically, in August of the same year, Garyth passed away and was not able to see all that has become of our work.

Determined to continue, I analyzed and published our original LMM study and continued to study both the vast amount of data as well as the work with the ultrasound as

biofeedback in the voice studio. Even so, the scope of its potential application was and still is not exhausted. Exploring my own tongue movements and the effect on the voice and working with my students—who have been an incredible help—I started to develop techniques and found indications to help master a more conscious and precise maneuvering/manipulation of the tongue.

I could not believe what I learned for my own singing and, by extension, as a pedagogue. I wished I would have had this tool and knowledge in my own study, cutting down a lot of explanations and—knowing now what is really happening—imaginary and even misguiding instructions. It is interesting that many voice users (including singers, actors, teachers, coaches, therapists, etc.) and scientists agree that the tongue is a crucial part in singing as well as speaking. Yet, there is no literature that solely addresses that organ and its acoustic influence in the context of a technique; in other words, what all does the tongue actually effect/influence? how can I manipulate/execute it for my purpose and why?

Of course, with the complexity of vocal production, it is never just one point that fixes everything. That said, the tongue is a major puzzle piece and should be, like breath support, posture, and so on, on the same checklist of fundamentals in voice production. By providing a visual demonstration of what is happening biomechanically and kinetically, students begin to feel the effect on the larynx as well as sensitize themselves to the possible physiological changes through muscle control and balance. This can help address, among other issues, the breathiness of a voice (vocal folds do not close because of tension in the tongue) and singing through the upper passaggio (transition into the top registers) with ease and without loss of timbre and intelligibility (often a result of tongue tension, tongue position—particularly for consonants and/or lack of pharyngeal resonance modification).

With the use of real-time video feedback and images derived from ultrasound, I observed a rapid acceleration in the students' understanding of complex vocal strategies that ultimately helps them to efficiently manifest a healthy vocal production in their own practice. No matter where I presented, gave workshops, or taught, it was the work with the ultrasound, and subsequently the attention on the tongue, that had the biggest effect. Statements like, "I cannot believe how important precise tongue positions are" or "I had no idea how much the tongue influences my voice" were not uncommon. This reality, plus the rapidly growing demand to have a book to refer to, and my excitement to help many vocal users by making this knowledge accessible, finally led me to write this book. It is by no means complete. The discoveries of new insight in the workings of the tongue, coupled with the acoustic influence and possible manipulations are ongoing. Even though I wanted the book to be as up-to-date as possible, I finally had to stop rewriting chapters every time I found something new. The primary audience for this book may be singers and actors, regardless of the level. Although based on scientific knowledge, it should not discourage those without a background in voice science. If anything, it should encourage them to get in touch with and maybe even become intrigued by it. For this reason, I tried not to omit technical terms, but I also did not make them a priority. Also, I purposely kept ancillary details to a minimum and simplified as much as possible. My focus in this book is the tongue and jaw. There are already multiple books and papers that cover vocal anatomy, physiology, and acoustics in great detail. Some of those "bibles" are referenced and should suffice—for those interested in more details and literature—to get off to a good start.

The book may also be useful to vocal therapists and professionals in related disciplines, giving a new perspective and ideas on vocal productions and analysis in everyday practice through the use of ultrasound. This may also be true for voice scientists. The spectrographic analysis on tongue shapes and various presented theories on consonants may be interesting for further research in the lab.

My research focus and goal is to make gained scientific knowledge and technological development more readily available and practically applicable to anyone who wants to learn how to sing or speak in a healthy manner and use the entire potential of their voice to express themselves. Since the "spectrographic big bang" in the evolution of voice pedagogy, many more books have been written by other authors who embrace the rapidly changing field of voice science and apply it in their pedagogical practice. Spectrography has since become a similar eye-body biofeedback that is now in extensive use in many voice studios worldwide.

I have been privileged and blessed by God to carry on Garyth's legacy together with him and now I am continuing and living it. So, it is my hope for the near future that ultrasound will follow the same path and find its way into the studios. Indeed, I am already working on development of an affordable USB transducer. Until then, I hope that this effort to codify new insights on tongue shapes and maneuvers will benefit all voice users and kindle new scientific studies, new appreciation for the complexity of voice production, new perspectives and ideas for voice pedagogy and therapy, and maybe even new excitement for voice research.

Note to the Reader

Many of the figure captions have two indicators for the color, e.g. gray/red. The first indicator refers to the black and white figure that appears in the printed book. The second refers to the full-color versions of the figures that can be found on the companion website.

For users of the eBook, the second color in the caption refers to the figures that appear within the book. There is no companion website access available for eBook users.

Acknowledgments

"Two are better than one [. . .]" (Ecclesiastes 4:9–12) is not only true in a marriage. Writing a book takes more than two people. In fact, I believe writing this book truly is a gift from God, who has chosen me as a conduit and has put many people into my life who had an impact on the outcome. Over the years, the numerous conversations I have had with teachers, mentors, colleagues, collaborators, students, allies, and friends have revised, confirmed, or inspired every word in this book. I would like to express my gratitude to all of you, and in particular to:

my mom for her unbroken support and love to me;

my dear friends Ginger, Eva Maria, Eva, Christopher, and Michi who made sure to help me keep my sanity through rough times (and there were plenty);

Dr. Mara Behlau for reading, mentoring, and supporting me throughout this process;

Rebecca Finkenauer, friend and colleague, for her reading in the early stages of the book;

Kathleen Bell, friend and voice researcher in her own right, for her invaluable feedback, continuous encouragement, and support of my work;

Anne Jacobson, for always being at the ready with guidance in the English language and any other matter;

Dr. Maureen Stone whose research of the tongue and vocal tract during speech, swallowing, and breathing using ultrasound is the cornerstone of my work—if it were not for her initial and generous support (taught me the use of ultrasound, provided the laboratory for initial studies) and mentoring throughout, none of this would have happened;

Dr. Bryan Gick for his collaboration as well as research that enriched my development of techniques for singing and resonant voice use;

my students for participating in this adventurous journey and for helping to explore the movements of the tongue and development of techniques;

Plural Publishing who saw the need to publish this book. Also, Valerie Johns and Christina Gunning who made sure of clarity and coherence with both professionalism and ethical sensitivity, as well as Lori Asbury, Jessica Bristow (Production), and Kristin Banach (Marketing); and

many, many more, who with their wisdom, knowledge, guidance, insight, support, and encouragement have made this book possible.

Reviewers

Plural Publishing and the author would like to thank the following reviewers for taking the time to provide their valuable feedback during the manuscript development process. Additional anonymous feedback was provided by other expert reviewers.

Corbin Abernathy, BM, MPerfA
The Vocal Actor with Corbin Abernathy
Instructor of Voice
Penn State Abington
Montgomery County, Pennsylvania

Thomas Bandy, DMA
Associate Professor of Collaborative
    Piano
Oberlin Conservatory of Music
Oberlin, Ohio

Kathleen Bell, BM, MM, DMA
Vocologist
Adjunct Instructor of Voice
Shenandoah University
Winchester, Virginia

Kaylene Cole, MM
Voice Teacher
West Palm Beach, Florida

Caroline Helton, DMA
Associate Professor of Music (Voice)
Department of Musical Theatre
University of Michigan School of Music,
    Theatre, and Dance
Ann Arbor, Michigan

Freda Herseth, BM, MM, HonDM
Arthur Thurnau Professor of Voice
University of Michigan School of Music,
    Theatre, and Dance,
Voice Training Specialist
Vocal Health Center
UM Health System
Ann Arbor, Michigan

Edrie Means Weekly, MM
Co-Founder
CCM Vocal Pedagogy Institute
Shenandoah University
Winchester, Virginia

In memory of my beloved late husband,
Garyth Nair

PART I

The Theory

1 It Is a Vowel-Centric World

Few of us ever stop to think about our ability to speak language—we speak every day, and each of us has been communicating in this way since we were between 12 and 18 months old. Our speech occurs automatically—we think a thought, and the words pour out without any conscious effort on our part. This automatic, background-processing nature of speech will take on huge significance later in this book when we begin to discuss high-level, classical singing in minute detail.

Singing Styles, Vocal Resonance, and Acting

This book is aimed to benefit all singers and actors alike, even though it is primarily geared to the high-level classical singer. Most singing styles, such as folk, pop, Broadway, and jazz (contemporary commercial music [**CCM**]), are **speech based**. This means that the phonemes of the language being sung are produced in almost the same manner as when the singer is speaking. In addition, the singer's voice is amplified, an often forgotten and, in its impact, underestimated component. Diction and intelligibility are still critical to the speech-based singer; achieving greater clarity is usually a matter of making sure that all the necessary pho-

nemes are present and sung with sufficient force to be heard.

However, classical singers do not operate in a speech-based world. The rich resonance that surrounds the language sounds of such singers differs significantly from their speech norms. This style also requires power sufficient enough to fill large venues without the aid of electrical amplification and to sing over the accompaniment of a full orchestra. This rich resonance creation is a learned behavior that takes *years* to develop properly. It must pervade all phonemes in the singer's output. This often presents a problem, because classical singers tend to concentrate far more on their vowel production than on that of their consonants; a subject that will be addressed in greater detail as we proceed.

You may ask, how does all of that correlate to acting? As mentioned earlier, in the speech-based singing style, sufficient force and presence seem to be enough in order to be heard. But the important puzzle piece for both **speech-based singing** and acting is *how* efficiently one is producing the force and presence. If you keep pushing and screaming from your throat (**larynx**) to get more power in your voice, you will not have much voice left after the premiere of the play. Frequently, such voice problems have already begun within the last few weeks before the premiere, when the intensity and frequency of rehearsals (and subsequently the voice abuse) increase, leaving actors little time to recuperate.

Although some of these circumstance in acting are similar to those in classical singing, it is interesting that so few actors seem to pay attention to how to use their voice properly in order to achieve good intelligibility and variety in their recitation. Many theaters lack good acoustics and/or are not supported by amplification. If speech-singing is not sufficient to carry a voice within those circumstances, why would a regular speech application do so? Just because one can speak does not mean that it is enough for the stage. That would be like saying that someone can play in the NFL simply because they can run and catch a football.

You may argue that this may not be as important in film and TV, where your voice is recorded through microphones and heavily processed by the sound engineer. I am aware of the trend toward a very natural way of speaking—aka "mumbling"—in those industries. But a BBC adaptation of *Jamaica Inn*, for instance, evoked hundreds of complaints from viewers who could not understand what the actors were saying, because they were so "natural" (in many cases, their thick accents were impenetrable). But do not take my word for it; Google the problem, and other films such as *Public Enemies*, *Shooter*, the *Pirates of The Caribbean* series, *Four Christmases*, *Miami Vice*, *The Wolfman*, *Be Kind Rewind*, *Fear and Loathing In Las Vegas*, and many Sylvester Stallone movies are quickly cited as examples.

Speech on stage has to be escalated over the speech norms we acquired since we are born, therefore requiring actors to be present more than the average 100%. When a singer starts to arrive at their first truly wonderful sung sounds, they are often reluctant to accept them as their own and describe

them as "fake" because it feels "foreign." The same is true for actors. The proof is easily shown with the **SAS ("say it as a singer")** exercise—the phrase was coined by Garyth Nair (1999, 2007)—in which the student is asked to *speak* the sounds of the phrase he or she is attempting to sing utilizing a *full, rich singing technique*.

To visualize our exercise, we use the **spectrogram** (Figure 1–1), a computer-generated analysis of sound that is extremely useful in both research and vocal study (Koenig, Dunn, & Lacy, 1946). The time is indicated from left to right, the **frequency** is indicated from bottom to top (the further up on the screen, the higher the frequency of the sound component), and the **loudness** is represented by the brightness of color of the graphic element. Of course, there is much more one can read in it, which we will do throughout the book, but for now that should suffice.

The graph in Figure 1–1 shows the Italian phrase, *Sospiri di foco, che l'aure in fiammate* performed three times: (a) spoken in a regular speech setting; (b) spoken with singer's resonance (utilizing the resonance of a classical technique); and (c) sung in classical style. The difference between the speech (first, left) and sung (third, right) is obvious. Interesting for us right now is the difference between the spoken (first, left) and the SAS (second, middle) phrases. In the latter, the singer speaks the phrase through the same vocal tract configuration used for singing. As a result, the vowels are showing much more harmonics (frequency) and loudness (brighter color) compared to the first one. It gets even more interesting when we look at the consonants (the core of this book, which we talk about in more detail later). Let us compare the first two vertical lines that indicate the consonants "s" and "sp" of *sospiri*. They show (a) more

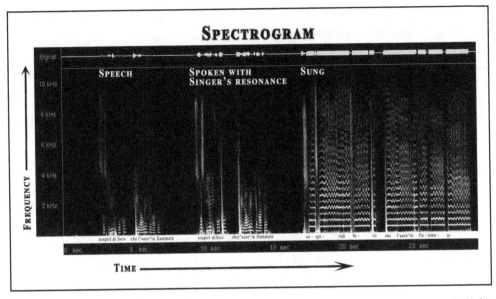

Figure 1–1. The phrase *Sospiri di foco, che l'aure in fiammate* performed as speech (*left*), speech utilizing the resonance of a classical technique (*middle*), and classical singing (*right*).

higher and lower frequencies, (b) more prominent and less scattered formants, and (c) increased intensity/loudness (brighter color). Thus, applying the singing technique in your speech leads to

- more resonance in all phonemes, vowels, and consonants;
- increased intelligibility because of purer phoneme-to-phoneme shifts; and
- an acoustical outcome that carries through any space, no matter the circumstances, while offering a variety of colors and dynamics for recitation.

The job of both singers and actors is to be a medium to convey a message through one of the greatest of all musical instruments: the human voice. We can only accomplish this with an effective delivery; for that, we have to train on how to use the body and learn the skills of voice/vocal use and body movement in the most efficient

and healthy way possible. This enables us to not only build the stamina for the entire performance (not just one aria/monologue) but also to sustain and carry through the circumambient demands such as stage/hall acoustics, accompaniment (orchestra, background noise, etc.), and much more.

This may sound like a lot of work, but the benefits of artistic excellence are for both artists and listeners. The audience's experience may run the whole gamut, from simply entertaining to total emotional transformation. Similarly, performers enjoy the personal fulfillment of performing great music/play, the physical and emotional excitement of making great sound (e.g., **endorphins**), the appreciation and validation from the audience, and so forth. As one of the great baritones, Thomas Hampson, once so beautifully said, "We don't present our voices to the audience, we resonate our souls."

Any discussion of singing or acting technique must deal with language in great specificity. In a very real sense, a high-level singer has to become a **phonetician**—one who deals with **phonetics,** the study of phonemes. Great singing, both in terms of tone and diction, depends on the singer's development of every needed phoneme to its fullest potential within his/her vocal technique.

> A **phoneme** is the basic building block of language; a singular, identifiable, and unique sound.

To illustrate, say the word "say" out loud but in slow motion so you can hear the individual sounds of the word (phonemes) one after the other. Notice that the long vowel is actually sounded with two phonemes: /e/ and /i/ (which are written in **International Phonetic Alphabet,** more on that later) so that the word would be written with the phonemes /s e i/. If we change the word to "see," even though the word is written with three letters, it only sounds as two phonemes: /s/ and /i/. When thinking of phonemes, it is critical to note that we are discussing individual sounds, not spelling. We can illustrate this by using the word itself: *phoneme.* The two written letters that begin the word, "ph," actually stand for a single phoneme, /f/. The entire word contains the phonemes /f o n i m/—five phonemes that took seven written letters to notate. As we go along, you will quickly learn this alphabet, and when you do, you will be on your way to being a better singer because you will be thinking in the language of sounds, not writing alphabets.

All languages are composed of two basic classes of phoneme:

- **Vowels**
- Consonants

As we see as we progress in this book, these two principal classes can be broken down into many subclasses (see Chapters 5, 6, and 7).

All singers speak during their everyday lives. In fact, we talk most of the time (when we are not singing). Thus, most of our interaction with language is through our speech, so speech seems to be a good place to begin our phonetic journey.

To illustrate some basic concepts, we are going to work with the same text used earlier from a famous song by the Baroque composer, Francesco Cavalli, *Sospiri di foco.* We use the first phrase of the song:

Sospiri di foco, che l'aure in fiammate

First, we must break down the component parts of the language (the phonemes), and we can see that this passage is composed of 29 separate phonemes (Figure 1–2). When we separate them by vowels versus consonants, we find that the passage is composed of a total of 15 vowels and 14 consonants distributed as shown in Figure 1–2.

When we speak the text of this passage, each of its 29 phonemes consumes a precise amount of time within the total 3.41 seconds (sec) that it takes to utter the entire passage. (We measure the execution time of each of the phonemes in milliseconds [msec, or thousandths of a second].) After

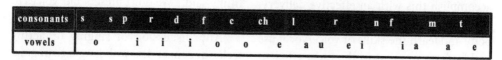

consonants	s	s	p	r	d	f	c	ch	l	r	n f	m	t
vowels	o	i	i	i	o	o	e	a u	e i	i a	a	e	

Figure 1–2. Cavalli, *Sospiri di foco*—consonant/vowel breakdown.

carefully measuring the length of each phoneme (using a spectrograph), we find that the execution time of the vowels totals 2.137 sec, and the total of the consonants equals 1.274 sec.

As you look at this distribution of vowels versus consonants in the graph in Figure 1–3, are you surprised at how close to equal their execution times are? Most people tend to think of languages in terms of vowels—another reason for our vowel-centricity.

This total phonemic execution time looks considerably different when we perform the same analysis on that text when sung according to Cavalli's musical notation (Figure 1–4). Now the total time for the sung phrase climbs to 8.28 sec, with the vowels consuming a whopping 6.72 sec (81%) of the total.

However, the total consonant execution time climbs only slightly as one can see in Figure 1–5.

When the data that produced the simple illustration in Figure 1–4 are recast to show execution times phoneme-to-phoneme, they produce the graph shown in Figure 1–6.

We now arrive at a critical point in this book.

This fact leads to a realization of why our singing culture is so vowel obsessed: because of composer's notation, the vowels are the phonemes that we sustain. They take up the lion's share of our time spent singing. Because of this time concentration, we have the luxury of concentrating on their production.

However, in singing, consonants fly by at roughly the same speed as they do in our speech. We do not have the same luxury of dwelling on their production because they are executed too fast. Because of this, the following occur:

- Singers *subconsciously* turn to *their automatic speech habits* for the neuromuscular instructions for their consonant production.
- While the resonance of our sung vowels is *exponentially greater* than those we produce in everyday speech, when we turn to our speech habits for consonant instructions, our consonants

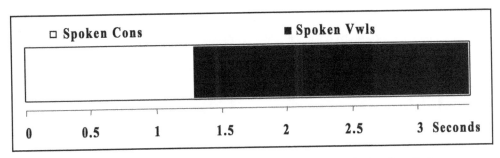

Figure 1–3. The execution time totals for vowels and consonants in the Cavalli phrase.

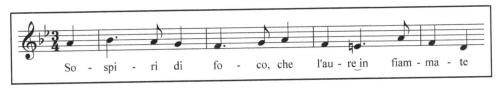

Figure 1–4. Cavalli, *Sospiri di foco*, opening phrase.

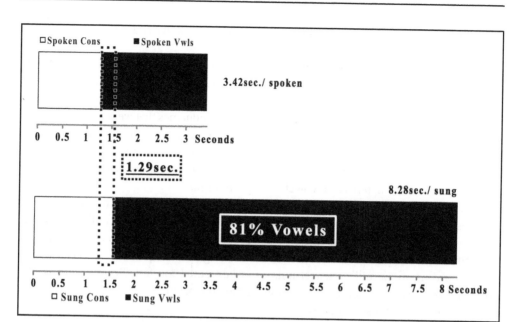

Figure 1–5. Vowel/consonant execution times—speech versus singing.

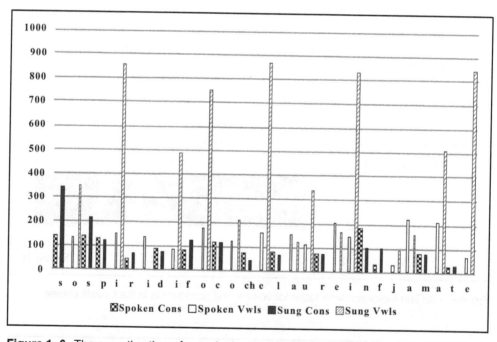

Figure 1–6. The execution times for each phoneme in the Cavalli text.

will be resonated as *far* less resonant phonemes.

■ During each speech-based consonant, the resonance spaces in the vocal tract collapse toward speech norms. There is simply no neurophysical means for the brain to be able to recover the full resonant space for the following vowel.

This leads us directly to the prime tenet of this book.

> **Great singers learn to produce CONSONANTS with a resonance that RIVALS their VOWELS.**

Once the singer has habituated appropriately resonant consonants, he/she is able to

- maintain the pharyngeal/oral space that produces the finest classical singing resonance *consistently* throughout the sung line, and
- once the consonants achieve this greater resonance, the diction of the singer instantly improves because these differently produced consonants will resound in the largest halls.

Now, we can also answer the question: Why don't my songs/monologues sound as good as my warm-ups?

Walk past any practice room when a singer-in-training is warming up on vowel vocalises (a melody sung only on vowels), and you may exclaim, "What a wonderful voice!" A few minutes later, when the same singer moves on to sing a song, you pass the room again, and it is as if another singer were there. The quality of the warm-up cannot be realized in the chaos of his/her attempts to toggle between singing vowels and spoken consonants. That is just another way of saying that all of the speech-based consonants are destroying the singer's ability to produce the very same vowels he or she was just singing during warm-up.

Now the reader knows why this book has been written. Any decent voice pedagogue can teach a student to sing vowels that he or she will be proud of. However, if that teacher never guides the student to concentrate on their consonant resonance (CR) with equal fervor, that singer may likely never realize the full potential of his other voice. The same is true for actors. In an age before microphones and cameras, the ability to project one's voice was an essential part of the classical theatrical repertoire. Any actor who mumbled would quickly have been booed off the stage. Nowadays, even on the cinema screen and in television, the consequences of that rigorous theatrical training are reflected in the precision of speech.

Throughout the history of singing, there have been teachers who have instinctively realized this technical need, going on to teach it to their students. By the same token, throughout history there have been singers who instinctively realized that their consonants deserved the same resonance as the vowels, and then went on to habituate a kind of resonance parity in their singing line. Whether it is the teacher, student, or a combination of both who works to impart equal resonance to both vowels and consonants, a great singer/actor is more than likely the result.

In this book, the secrets of CR will be revealed. This is no new discovery—singers who know this "secret" have sung among us for as long as *bel canto* has existed. Laurence Olivier, Sean Connery, Morgan Freeman, Meryl Streep, Judi Dench, Ingrid Bergman, and Helen Mirren are just a few examples of actors whose formal training stressed perfect diction in order to be taken seriously.

All we need to do is look and listen (YouTube has become a goldmine for this kind of study), and we can see that great singers and actors are demonstrating these techniques right out in the open. This book attempts to guide you in your discovery of these "secrets" so you can join their ranks.

So, now, let us explore the *Secret Life of Consonants*.

References

Koenig, W., Dunn, K., & Lacy, L. Y. (1946). The sound spectrograph. *Journal of the Acoustical Society of America, 18,* 19–49.

Nair, G. (1999). *Voice, tradition and technology.* San Diego, CA: Singular Publishing.

Nair, G. (2007). *The craft of singing.* San Diego, CA: Plural Publishing.

2 Anatomy and Physiology

An exploration of the nature of sung or spoken sounds calls for an understanding of anatomy and physiology of the human body. For singers and actors who want to improve their skills, it is indispensable to have an understanding of not only vocal production but also the mechanism of the articulators and tongue, respectively. Additionally, body mechanics, such as those of head, neck, and jaw, are built on proper body posture. In this chapter, we mainly explore anatomical and biomechanical principles as they apply to the mechanism of the articulators and tongue. If you would like to know more about the voice production itself, there is much literature available on this subject. Some examples are Miller (1986), Nair (2007), *Oxford Handbook of Singing* (2019), Sundberg (1989), Titze (2000), and Titze and Verdolini-Abbott (2012).

Anatomical Terminology

Some anatomical terms may usefully be revisited for a better understanding and discussion of basic body structures. In an anatomical sense, humans are always described in the upright (erect) position with eyes looking forward. The upper limbs are at the sides of the body with the palms facing forward; it is called the anatomical position.

Directional Planes

Directional planes refer to the two-dimensional sections of the body as follows (Figure 2–1):

Sagittal—dividing the body into left and right;

Frontal (coronal)—dividing the body into front and back (anterior and posterior or ventral and dorsal); and

Transverse—dividing the body into head and tail (cranial and caudal).

Directional Terms

These terms describe the positions of structures relative to other structures or locations in the body (Figure 2–2):

Anterior—structures toward the front of the body;

Posterior—structures toward the back of the body;

Superior—above another part of the body;

Inferior—below another part of the body;

Medial—position closer to the midline or center of the body (e.g., the middle toe is located at the medial side of the foot);

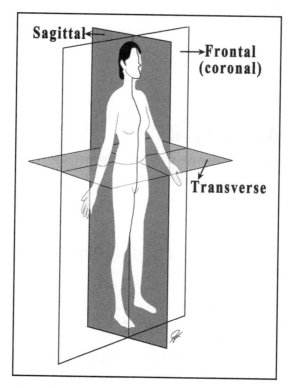

Figure 2–1. Commonly used anatomical directional planes.

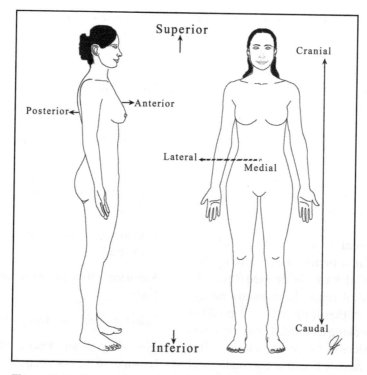

Figure 2–2. Commonly used anatomical directional terms.

Lateral—position away from the midline or center of the body (e.g., the little toe is located at the lateral side of the foot);

Cranial—toward the skull of the body; and

Caudal—toward the bottom of the body.

The Mandible

The mandible is the largest, strongest, and lowest bone in the face (Standring & Gray, 2008). Its structure consists of the

body—the curved, somewhat horseshoe-like shape holding the lower teeth in place;

ramus (or rami, plural for both sides)— the perpendicular part of the mandible and connects to the skull; and

angle—where the body and ramus connect (Figure 2–3).

The two protrusions at the top of the ramus connect the mandible to the skull as follows:

The coronoid process—This is the smaller, thinner, and more anterior (front) protrusion, connecting to the temporalis muscle.

The condyle—This is the larger, thicker, and more posterior (back) protrusion, connecting to the temporal bone of the skull.

The joint where the mandible and temporal bone meet is called the temporomandibular joint (TMJ). The TMJ is one of the most complex joints in the body, providing hinging and gliding movements at the same

time. Figure 2–4 shows how the articular disc separates the condyle from the mandibular fossa. Between the condyle and the disc is the inferior joint cavity. This is also where the first part of the mouth opening occurs via pure rotation of the condyle.

Exterior Laryngeal Muscles

What stands out in Figure 2–3 is the seemingly free-floating hyoid bone. Unlike other bones that are in close proximity, the hyoid is only distantly articulated to other bones by muscles or ligaments, rendering its primary function as an anchor for the tongue. For example, when the hyoglossus (see Figure 2–7, later in the chapter) on both sides contracts to depress the tongue and widen the oral cavity, the hyoid bone anchors them. The same is true below (inferior), connecting it to the sternum, clavicle, and scapula (shoulder). This anchoring structure (Figure 2–5) can be likened to docking a vessel (the hyoid bone) by tying it "fore and aft" (the muscles above and below the hyoid bone) to keep it both floating and secure and steady.

Most of the explanations of the means by which the larynx is lowered focus on the action of the laryngeal depressor muscles. You can see we have two groups of muscles below (infra) and above (supra) the hyoid bone, and they are connected directly or indirectly to it. Hence, the names infrahyoid (beneath the hyoid) and suprahyoid (above the hyoid) muscles. The infrahyoid muscles (or strap muscles) are the depressor muscles responsible for lowering the larynx. These four strap muscles are as follows:

Sternohyoid—This connects the upper part of the sternum, manubrium, with the hyoid bone.

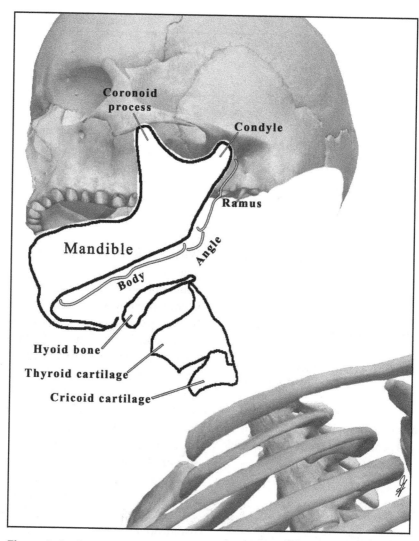

Figure 2–3. Sagittal anatomical structures referenced in this chapter.

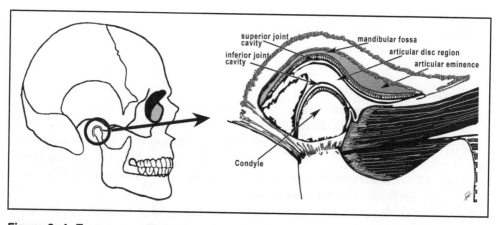

Figure 2–4. Temporomandibular joint (TMJ): between the inferior and superior joint cavities (*green*) is the articular disc (*white*) that separates the condyle from the mandibular fossa.

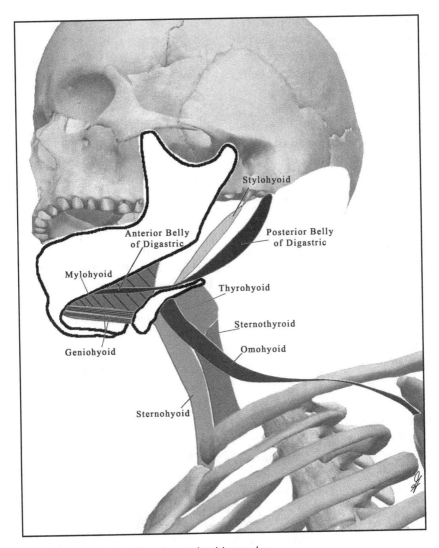

Figure 2–5. Infrahyoid and suprahyoid muscles.

Omohyoid—This consists of two segments, bellies, that are linked through an intermediate tendon on the clavicle. The superior belly connects to the hyoid bone, and the inferior belly connects to the scapula.

Sternothyroid—This connects the upper part of the sternum, manubrium, with the thyroid cartilage.

Thyrohyoid—This links the thyroid and hyoid (*note:* this muscle can either raise the larynx or lower the hyoid).

The suprahyoid (upper) muscles are responsible for the elevation of the larynx, and in comparison to the rather similarly formed infrahyoid (lower) muscles, the shape of the suprahyoid muscles is quite different. These four muscles, which can be seen in Figure 2–5, are as follows:

Digastric—As with the omohyoid, this muscle consists of two bellies, which are connected at an intermediate tendon on the hyoid bone. The **anterior belly** of the digastric arises from a depression of the inner side of the lower border of the mandible, while the longer **posterior belly** of the digastric arises from the mastoid process (you can feel a protuberance on the border of the skull behind the ear).

Stylohyoid—This arises from the styloid process (just anteriorly from the mastoid process) and connects the hyoid bone.

Mylohyoid—This is a triangular, flat, and thin muscle that forms a sling inferior to the tongue building the floor beneath it on both left and right sides. It arises from the inside of the mandible (*mylohyoid line*) and inserts into the hyoid bone.

Geniohyoid—Similar to the mylohyoid, the geniohyoid is a paired, narrow muscle. It arises from the inner surface of the chin (Latin *genio* is the prefix for "chin") and inserts into the hyoid bone.

The Tongue

The tongue is quite a unique part in our body. It is interesting that its musculature structure is only comparable to that of the heart. Both are entirely composed of soft tissue; however, the tongue normally moves about 10 times faster, and the muscle architecture, as you will soon see, is considerably more complex than the heart.

Now imagine that you have a tube around 16 cm in length in which you put in a portion of Play-Dough (a modeling compound used for arts and crafts) about

9 cm in size—the average size of the tongue (Sanders, Mu, Amirali, Su, & Sobotka, 2013). You would very quickly see that this Play-Dough occupies more than half of the tube. Translate this image to the vocal tract (VT), and it becomes almost a no-brainer that the tongue is one of the major active articulators within the VT (Figure 2–6).

Before I started to specialize in the **physioacoustics** of the tongue through ultrasound, I never appreciated how large of a muscle it actually is. Since we cannot see the tongue in its entirety, it is very tempting to believe that the tongue consists only of the part that one can stick out. However, have a look at Figure 2–7, and you can see that this visible part (labeled as tongue) is only a fraction of all the muscles it is composed of.

This fascinating muscular organ is considered a muscular hydrostat that consists only of muscles and has no skeletal support. The latter means that the musculature itself both creates movement and provides skeletal support for that movement. As if this is not interesting enough, in addition, one of the most important biomechanical features of a hydrostat is that it is volume preserving. What does that mean? Imagine a water balloon: no matter how you squeeze, dent, or pinch it, only the shape and/or surface will change, while the volume will always stay the same. Thus, a compression in one location means an expansion in at least one other dimension (Kier & Smith, 1985; Smith & Kier, 1989).

Before we move forward in this book— and in the interest of the quest for expanding and updating our knowledge, so vocal myths can be dispelled and averted in order to prevent singers/actors from misguided advice—I would like to emphasize and ask to keep in mind this important characteristic of a muscular hydrostat, particularly in terms of instructions on the tongue's move-

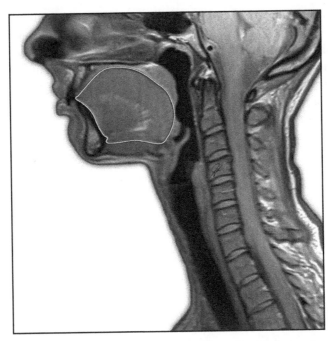

Figure 2–6. Midsagittal magnetic resonance image: tongue at rest (*red contour*). Courtesy of Medical University of Graz, Austria.

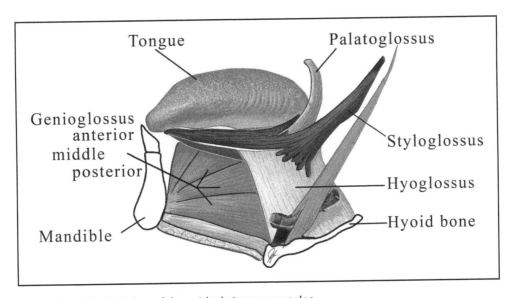

Figure 2–7. Sagittal view of the extrinsic tongue muscles.

ment and position (kinesthetics), a matter of "perception versus physiology" (Chapter 5). As I stated in the preface, I wished I would have had this knowledge and tool (ultrasound) in my own study, cutting down a lot of explanations and, more importantly, imaginary and misguiding instructions. It is not uncommon to hear teachers, coaches, and others guide with instructions such as, "move the tongue forward," "move the tongue back," or "put the tip up." However, in the context of the muscular hydrostat, these instructions are rather misguided and even counterproductive. Why? Because, as mentioned earlier, a muscular hydrostat means that *every movement* of the tongue is accompanied by *deformation*. For example, if you move the tip (apex) of the tongue, the entire tongue has to move, thus resulting in a reshaping of the whole tongue because the volume is constant. In Chapter 6 we introduce even more details of the tongue's complexity, particularly three-dimensionally, and how segments of the tongue move in opposite directions. While with the categories of front and back vowels it is very tempting to say "move your tongue back" for an /ɑ/ (as in l<u>a</u>w). However, as you will see, it is a reshaping of the tongue where the front is compressed and the back is elongated, thereby resulting in more tongue volume in the throat (pharyngeal) area rather than the entire tongue pushed backward.

With this in mind, let us have a look at this composition of tongue muscles. The tongue is the only part of our body that is able to simultaneously retract and extend. This is possible because of the muscles of the tongue that can be classified as either **extrinsic** (outside) or **intrinsic** (inside) (see Figure 2–7).

Characteristic of the **extrinsic tongue muscles** is that they are linked to surrounding bones and tissues. Their main function is to alter the position of the tongue (through vertical and horizontal movements) as well as produce quite complicated tongue surface shapes, which help in the making of vowel sounds (see Chapter 4).

The extrinsic muscles include the following:

Palatoglossus (PG)—This attaches only soft structures to other soft structures and forms the lowest muscular layer of the soft palate, connecting the velum to the tongue below. Arising from the anterior surface of the soft palate, the PG proceeds downward and forward into the side of the tongue and can either depress and/or raise the velum.

Hyoglossus (HG)—This attaches the side of the tongue to the hyoid bone. Connecting the superior border of the hyoid bone with the side of the tongue, the HG depresses the tongue down and back.

Styloglossus (SG)—This rises from the styloid processes (a downward pointed piece of bone from the temporal bone of the skull, just below the ear) downward and forward. Running along the side of the tongue, the SG divides into two parts, one running intertwined along the inferior longitudinal muscle (see intrinsic muscles) and the other merging/overlapping with the HG.

Genioglossus (GG)—This rises like a hand fan at the midline from the mandible and protrudes and depresses the tongue. Proportional to the other muscles, the GG forms the majority of the body of the tongue, and its contractions will pull the midline tongue inward, producing a midline groove (see Chapters 4 and 6). Furthermore, it can be controlled independently, producing a groove in one place but not another. These different actions are controlled by three major regions in the GG:

- **genioglossus anterior** (GGa) lowers and retracts the front of the tongue,
- **genioglossus middle** (GGm) lowers the tongue body and pulls it forward, and

■ **genioglossus posterior** (GGp) pulls the tongue root forward when contracted.

The other group of muscles within the tongue includes the **intrinsic tongue muscles** that both originate and insert within the tongue, running along the tongue. In contrast to the extrinsic tongue muscles, these muscles are not attached to any bone and act to alter the shape of the tongue (Figure 2–8). Four bilateral muscles provide an internal flexibility (essential to the formation of consonants when complex shapes and rapid changes in shape and position are required). These four muscles can be paired into the following:

Superior longitudinal (SL) and **inferior longitudinal muscles**

(IL)—These muscles run lengthwise front-to-back through the tongue and connect the anterior and posterior ends. Contracting the SL muscle curls the apex (tip) of the tongue upward. The IL runs along either side of the genioglossus and helps give the tongue a convex shape.

Verticalis and **transversus muscles**— These muscles are interwoven. The verticalis is located in the middle of the tongue and connects the superior and inferior surfaces vertically. The transversus muscles run horizontally, connecting the left and right sides.

The contractions of these intrinsic muscles will alter the shape of the tongue by bringing the two attached sides closer together, as

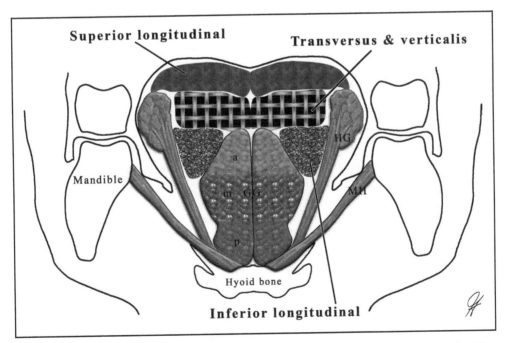

Figure 2–8. Coronal cross section of the tongue. The intrinsic tongue muscles are paired like a sandwich, with the superior and inferior longitudinal muscles as the slices of bread and the transversus and verticals being the peanut butter and jelly in the middle. Note how the indicated hyoglossus (HG), mylohyoid (MH), and genioglossus (GG) are connected to a bone structure (hyoid, mandible) and building the foundation for the intrinsic muscles.

well as by shortening and lengthening, widening (flattening) and narrowing (rounding) it, and curling and uncurling the edges and apex.

Both extrinsic and intrinsic tongue muscles are well orchestrated for the production of vowels and consonants. However, by slowly putting the puzzle pieces presented here together, there is one more rather important aspect—one of the reasons for writing this book—that has to be taken into account: the **low mandible maneuver** (LMM).

Because the extrinsic tongue muscles are connected to bones, any movement of the mandible automatically effects the position of the tongue. This, in turn (whether in speaking or singing), ultimately has an effect on both the phoneme and the sound resonance. We continue to discuss the effect of the LMM on the tongue and resonance, respectively, in more detail in the next chapter.

Antagonism

Before moving to the next chapter, I would like to conclude by touching on a subject that, in my opinion, should always be kept in mind when talking about anatomy and physiology.

The entire body is a fascinating though extremely complex *Gesamtkunstwerk* (total work of art). The deeper one looks into the body's physiology, the harder it becomes to simplify the understanding of the mechanism—or even control it, for that matter. Of course, the latter is of particular interest for us, since we want to develop a new habit and be able to access it on command. But it seems as if there is never just *one* way or mechanism that any movement of

our body is based on. For instance, all the muscles above the hyoid bone (suprahyoid muscles) mentioned earlier are connected to the hyoid bone, which is why their contraction results in elevation of the larynx. You might now ask why muscles that generally elevate the hyoid bone and in turn the larynx are important for a laryngeal drop and pharyngeal elongation? The two muscle groups—infrahyoid and suprahyoid—work in concert antagonistically. Such muscle antagonism is what gives us control over almost everything we do. This is especially true in the symphony of muscular interaction needed to produce accurate, precise, and resonant pitches. It would be beyond the scope of this book to get into every detail. However, being equipped with the basic principles and some supporting contextual thoughts of physiology and statics should help avoid any excessive, unnecessary force—especially in beginners—while trying to execute certain tasks, such as dropping or keeping down the jaw.

When we look at the two muscle groups (Figure 2–9), it is not unlike a tug-of-war (two teams pulling on opposite ends of the rope) where the team "infrahyoid muscles" is pulling on one side and the team "suprahyoid muscles" is pulling on the other, with the hyoid bone as the "center line." The goal of the game is to bring the center line a certain distance in one direction against the force of the opposing team's pull. In our case, it would be lowering the hyoid bone. However, unlike tug-of-war, the object is not to have one team pulling over the other. Rather, we want to have both teams balancing the ratio of their force (one muscle group [agonist] versus the other [antagonist]) depending on the demands and task. This means keeping the hyoid bone in such a way that it maintains a lowered, yet relaxed position or providing the flexibility for it to

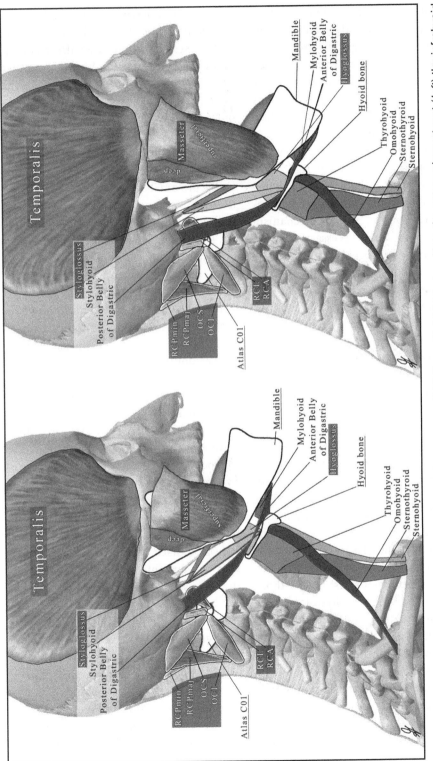

Figure 2–9. Major muscles involved in the low mandible maneuver (LMM): sagittal (side) view. Note the antagonism: at rest (*left*) the infrahyoid muscles are relaxed/stretched, whereas the suprahyoid as well as the two major chewing muscles (temporalis and masseter) are contracted. With the applied LMM (*right*), the depressor muscles (infrahyoid muscles) are contracted (lowering the larynx) and the jaw elevators (temporalis, masseter, suprahyoid muscles) need to relax/expand so the condyle smoothly translates along the articular eminence.

tilt without cementing one muscle group into place. It is this sensitive control of the rate, direction, and force of the preparatory movement that is necessary to execute a delicate task, such as timbral variations or resonant, pitch-producing action (which is why it is extremely difficult to design and build a machine to do similar delicate tasks).

The previously mentioned example seems to appear simple enough, right? Two groups of muscles on each side, balancing contraction and relaxation. Although simplifying and focusing on that mechanism is certainly a good and necessary start, we must keep in mind that this is just one side of the equation or, better yet, one gear in an intricate clock mechanism. We have not even looked at the intrinsic muscles attached within the larynx or at the head and neck muscles.

In spite of this, it is the antagonism that I wanted to draw attention to, and that is particularly important to bear in mind, since voice pedagogues, coaches, actors, and singers are quick to judge or repudiate certain "techniques"—such as the LMM—because it may turn into a counterproductive tightening of the pharynx, TMJ, or any other crucial part in our voice production. However, it is extremely difficult, particularly for beginners, to immediately control the symphony of muscles involved in voice production. As in any movement of the body, it is imperative to first have a thorough understanding of physiology and then slowly learn to build a database of neuromuscular activations, combining the nervous system (neuro) and the muscular system (muscular).

Yet again, looking at antagonism through the skeleton musculature is only one part of the equation. There is no doubt that isolating a single muscle and analyzing its function, by determining what would happen if the two ends are approximated, makes it easier to understand the complexity of muscle function in general. However, the skeletal system of our body also has **ligaments** (connecting one bone to another bone), **tendons** (connecting muscle to the bone), and **fasciae** (connecting muscles to other muscles), among other fibrous layers. These are the reasons, among others, why one muscle could have a huge effect on its neighbor—not to mention any influence on the proximal or distal structures beyond it—by, for instance, tightening its fascia or pushing against it.

This is important to keep in mind when one talks about muscle contraction, relaxation, or the like when working on things like posture, support, LMM, tongue positions, and so forth. For example, too often, especially when working with beginners, a lot of force is applied to drop and/or keep the jaw down. This can be counterproductive to achieving the actual goal of subsequent relaxed pharyngeal lengthening/laryngeal drop.

The biomechanics of the mandible elevation (rise) and depression (drop), the tongue, as well as the TMJ, is a finely tuned dynamic balance among all head and neck muscles. Looking at the entire body from the perspective of geometry—like an architecture of muscles as well as fasciae and not only as a stack of bones—helps circumvent any unwanted laryngeal tension and therefore support an open and relaxed tone production.

Through that perspective, the term *tensegrity* comes to mind. Coined by the famous architect, Richard Buckminster Fuller, it is a portmanteau of "tension + integrity." The concept behind it is best depicted by the model in Figure 2–10. You can see how the integrity of the structure is derived from the balance of tension members and not the compression of struts. Traditionally, the integrity of most buildings

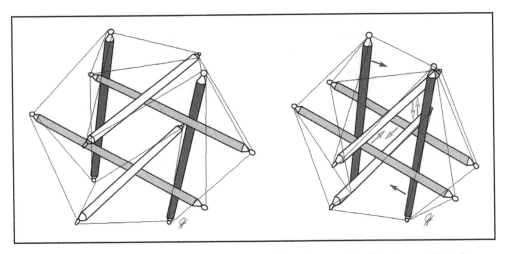

Figure 2–10. Model showing the structural principle of tensegrity. The bones (struts), connected through the myofasciae (elastic bands), give the structure strength and flexibility. One would think that pressing the dark gray/red struts together would push the others apart. However, that is not the case. Any strain (push or pull) will always be distributed throughout the structure in one direction, resulting in an expansion or contraction of the entire model (like the body). Hence, the balance between bones and myofascia always works in a one-directional movement. Try it out and build your own tensegrity model. You will find a lot of instructions on YouTube: it is fun and fascinating.

and houses lies on the integrity of continuous compression, starting from the highest to the lowest brick. Too often, our body is thought of in the same way: the skeleton is a stack of bones (continuous compression) that are moved by the muscles hanging off each bone. However, as previously mentioned, our skeleton is surrounded by soft tissue. This myofascial network is like an adjustable tensegrity around the skeleton: imagine a grid of elastics that, like the struts in the tensegrity model, keep the bones in place or move them through a continuous inward pulling tension, while maintaining an overall strength/intensity (Myers, 2014). However, for the sake of simplicity, we continue to use the term "muscle" only, though with the knowledge now that the fasciae are part of the functional connection.

So, no matter what the movement in our body, we should be very careful not to exacerbate it by pushing, tightening, or overstretching muscles just for the sake of making it work. This is important to keep in mind—particularly within the context of *tensegrity*—because, as in the physiology of LMM, the goal is to put "strain" into the structure (dropping the jaw and keeping it in place), while letting the deformation be distributed consistently throughout the head and neck, so their finely tuned dynamic muscles are able to work together and not inhibit each other (see Figure 2–10). Other mechanisms, such as support, work in the same way. One cannot just contract the abdominal muscles and expect to have the reflective reaction (subsequently, control) over the diaphragm. It is again what I like to call a "flexible contraction" made to accommodate the miniscule changes occurring on every single pitch or dynamic change. And let us not forget the co-contraction (occurring in the back of the body), which is the simultaneous contraction of agonist and antagonist to maintain, for example, stability of the diaphragm. Please bear in mind that this is grossly simplified and may well become the subject of another book. However, it is one of the biomechanical principles that has served in my studio and in my approach to voice technique and body alignment extremely successfully for over a decade.

To round it off a bit more, let us have a little more fun using another example of anatomy and physiology at work. Have I mentioned how complex our body is? As you can see in Figures 2–11 and 2–12, we

have another group, namely, the short neck muscles—**suboccipital muscles**—where we have a tremendous neurological input and which attach to either the C1 (atlas) or C2 (axis) vertebrae. All of them together rock and tilt the head into extension, and some assist in the rotation of the head. In addition, these muscles play a critical role in stabilization and fine movement control of the cranium on the atlas, and the atlas on the axis. Putting this muscle group into the same context of antagonism and tensegrity,

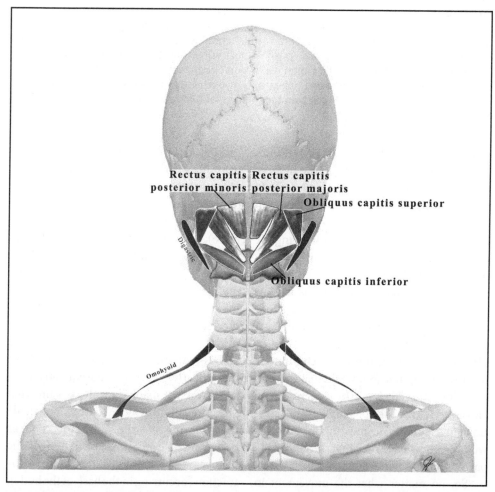

Figure 2–11. Posterior (back) view of the suboccipital muscles. Note the darker/dark red indicates digastric (infrahyoid muscle) and omohyoid (suprahyoid muscle) showing how each body part is connected with the other.

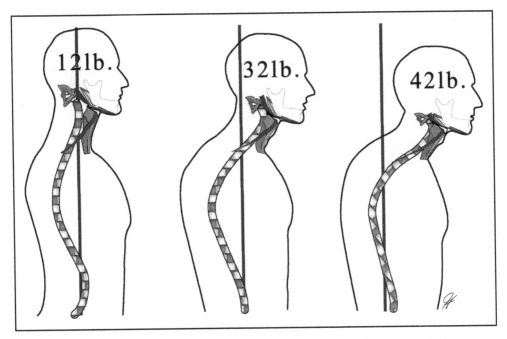

Figure 2–12. For every inch of forward head motion, the head's weight increases by 10 pounds. Also, note how the integrity of every muscle group (short neck muscles, infrahyoid and suprahyoid muscles) becomes more contracted, hence putting constant strain on them and preventing links like temporomandibular joint, hyoid bone, skull and spine (C1 and C2), thorax, and so forth from moving freely and working properly.

you will quickly see why they are important for the LMM, for a relaxed laryngeal position, for breathing or for the entire posture, for that matter.

According to Kapandji (1974), for every inch the head moves forward, it gains 10 pounds in weight (see Figure 2–12). To prevent the head (chin) from dropping onto the chest, the upper back and neck muscles (**trapezius** and **levator scapula**) have to work much harder, while the anterior (front) and opposing musculature tightens and shortens (**pectoralis major** and **minor**). As a result, we are confronted with an "upper crossed syndrome," first noted by Vladimir Janda (1988). Furthermore, according to Rene Cailliet, the **forward head motion** (FHM) and the resultant loss of the inward curvature of the spine (**cervical lordosis**) will block the infrahyoid muscles—also respon-

sible for helping to lift the first rib during inhalation—in particular, which may result in the loss of some 30% of vital lung capacity. Additionally, Hack et al. (1985) have found a connective tissue bridge between the rectus capitis posterior minor muscle and the outermost membrane covering the spinal cord and brain (**dura mater**). Hence, with a forward head motion, the short neck muscles remain in constant contraction, putting pressure on the nerve and possibly causing headaches at the base of the skull.

There is much more to write on this topic, but for now, I would refer you to the article by Wright et al. (2009) as well as the book by J. P. Okeson (2012), both of which will get you started and guide you through the complex though fascinating world of the fasciae. The next stop for us will be the principles of resonance creation.

References

Hack G. D., Koritzer, R. T., Robinson, W. L., Hallgren, R. C., Greenman, P. E. (1995). Anatomic relation between the rectus capitis posterior minor muscle and the dura mater. *Spine, 20*(23), 2484–2486.

Janda, V. (1988). Muscles and cervicogenic pain syndromes. In R. Grand (Ed.), *Physical therapy of the cervical and thoracic spine* (pp. 153–166). New York, NY: Churchill Livingstone.

Kapandji, I. A. (1974). *The physiology of the joints: Vol. 3. The trunk and the vertebral column* (L. H. Honor, Trans.). Edinburgh, UK: Churchill Livingstone.

Kier, W. M., & Smith, K. K. (1985). Tongues, tentacles and trunks: The biomechanics of movement in muscular-hydrostats. *Zoological Journal of the Linnean Society, 83*, 307–324.

Miller, R. (1986). *The structure of singing*. New York, NY: Schirmer.

Myers, T. W. (2014). *Myofascial meridians for manual and movement therapists* (3rd ed.). New York, NY: Elsevier, Churchill Livingstone.

Nair, G. (2007). *The craft of singing*. San Diego, CA: Plural Publishing.

Okeson, J. P. (2012). *Management of temporomandibular disorders and occlusion* (7th ed.). St. Louis, MO: Mosby.

Sanders, I., Mu, L., Amirali, A., Su, H., & Sobotka, St. (2013). The human tongue slows down to speak: Muscle fibers of the human tongue. *Anatomical Record, 296*(10), 1615–1627.

Smith, K. K., & Kier, W. M. (1989). Trunks, tongues, and tentacles: Moving with skeletons of muscle. *American Scientist, 77*, 28–35.

Standring, S., & Gray, H. (2008). *Gray's anatomy. The anatomical basis of clinical practice* (40th ed.). New York, NY: Churchill Livingstone/ Elsevier.

Sundberg, J. (1987). *The science of the singing voice*. Dekalb, IL: Northern Illinois University Press.

Titze, I. (2000). *Principles of voice production* (2nd ed.). Iowa City, IA: National Center for Voice and Speech.

Titze, I., & Verdolini-Abbott, K. (2012). *Vocology: The science and practice of voice habilitation*. Salt Lake City, UT: National Center for Voice and Speech.

Welch, G. F., Howard, D. M., & Nix, J. (Eds.). (2019). *Oxford handbook of singing*. Oxford, UK: Oxford University Press.

Wright, E. F., & North, S. L. (2009). Management and treatment of temporomandibular disorders: A clinical perspective. *The Journal of Manual & Manipulative Therapy, 17*(4), 247–254. https://doi.org/10.1179/10669810979135 2184

3 Principles of Resonance Creation—The Low Mandible Maneuver

We singers/speakers have a **semienclosed airspace resonator** or **semioccluded vocal tract** (SOVT), as well as the only continuously malleable resonator in music (Figure 3–1).

Because we can change our resonance spaces in so many ways, we are able to produce a remarkable variety of tone colors and, most importantly, produce (spoken) language. There are many books that cover those subjects in greater depth. The interested reader may consult Howard & Murphy (2008), Nair (2007), Sataloff (2005), Sundberg (1989), and Titze (1994). For the contextual interest of this book, we only briefly review some parts and, where necessary, introduce new ones and elaborate on others in more detail.

Acoustics

All singers/speakers are wind instruments. Utilizing the oboe as an exemplar, all of the component parts for the creation of sound are shared by both instruments (Table 3–1).

The difference in Table 3–1 that is most important for us, and which is at the core of this book, is the singer designation for resonator—**highly malleable resonator shapes—pharynx and oral cavity.**

What does that mean? A sound generator produces sound energy that vibrates in sympathy with a **resonator,** found in almost all musical instruments. This resonator is placed between the sound source and the conveying medium (air) and can either be an object, or space that has resonance. Unlike the tone generator, resonators do not impart energy to the atmosphere but react to and vibrate with the generated sound. A great example of this is the phenomenon of a singer shattering glass. If you gently flick the glass, you can hear the frequency of the glass. When you match this frequency and increase the volume to its maximum, the glass will start to vibrate until it breaks. Some of those vibrations may not be visible to the naked eye without a slow-motion camera. However, just go on YouTube, and you will find numerous videos that show a variety of examples.

Resonators

We differentiate between two different types of resonators:

- The **general** or **forced resonator** is where the vibrations of the tone generator are conveyed to a resonating

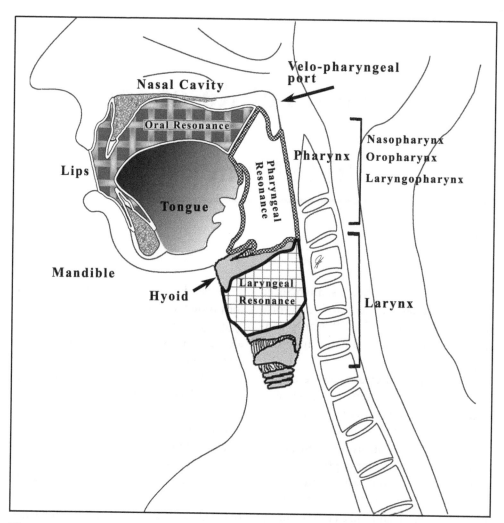

Figure 3–1. Sagittal view of the resonance spaces of the vocal system.

Table 3–1. Comparison of the Sound Creation Elements of an Oboe and a Singer		
Sound Creation Elements	*Oboe*	*Singer/Speaker*
Energy supply	Player's respiratory system	Singer's respiratory system
Tone generator	Reed	Vocal folds in the larynx
Variable pitches	Holes on the resonator that vary the air column length	Accomplished by varying the tension on the vocal fold length (muscles)
Resonator	Fixed resonator—body of the instrument, conical and made of hard wood	Highly malleable resonator shapes—the space above larynx (pharynx) and mouth (oral cavity)
Bell—where the resonator interacts with the environment	Small flared aperture at the end of the resonator	Mouth

material. For instance, the soundboard of a piano reacts with vibrations to the activated strings (source) and, thus, reinforces the sound by presenting a larger vibrating surface to the atmosphere. This type of resonator is making the transfer of sound far more efficient.

- The **semienclosed airspace** is the type of resonator that also most closely approximates the model of the human voice: a tube. Closed at one end and open at the other, it is like a column of air in a cylinder. We find this type of resonator in all woodwind and brass instruments. The closed end consists of the lips, reeds, and other parts, and the open end is commonly called the **bell**.

Let us have a look at the oboe again. The instrument has a conical-shaped resonator coupled with a tone generator consisting of a double reed (two pieces of vibrating cane kept in motion by the oboist's breath energy). Playing a pitch on the reed alone will show some harmonic peaks on the spectra (plural of spectrum; Chapters 1, 5, and 7). However, if you play the same pitch attached to the resonator, the spectra will

show the same harmonic peaks but with a greater amplitude (Figure 3–2).

This is because the sound waves start to travel from the closed end to the open end where they will bounce, reflect off (echo) (sound is able to reflect off even on an open end: air pressure is above and below atmospheric pressure, so the wave reflects off the open end because of a compression turning into an expansion). That returning echo will meet with the sound source again, and once they match, they will amplify each other (Figure 3–3).

The Low Mandible Maneuver

Most singers eventually achieve the optimally open mouth. In their vowel production, most also become adept at lowering their larynx.

However, it is the low mandible maneuver (LMM) (Nair, Nair, & Reishofer, 2016) that is usually the missing link in singers' techniques. This last element, found abundantly in the technique of singers of international rank, if learned and habituated, frees

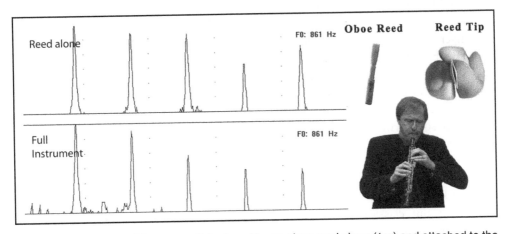

Figure 3–2. Spectra of the same pitch played by an oboe reed alone (*top*) and attached to the instrument (resonator) (*bottom*). (Spectra image from *The Craft of Singing* [p. 173] by Garyth Nair © 2007 Plural Publishing. All Rights Reserved.)

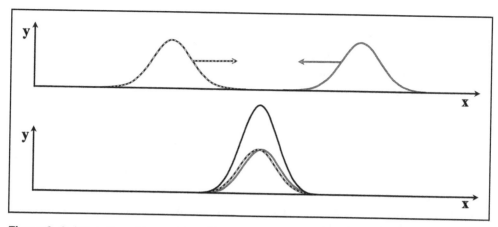

Figure 3–3. Interaction of two waves, with equal frequency and magnitude, traveling in opposite directions (*top*). Once the waves meet and match, they amplify each other (*bottom*).

the voice to its finest production. The reason why this is helpful for actors/actresses is once again, variety. Being able to maneuver and open the jaw while reciting can give more intensity and tone. Screaming on stage, also often the substitute for loudness, will be exhausting and damage the vocal folds if not done in a healthy manner. You will soon see that being able to maneuver all active articulators (see Chapter 4), including the jaw, will enable you to project better and be more efficient without strain.

Now, do you remember the warm-up story in Chapter 1? Because most warm-ups are vocalises involving only vowels, the singer's vocal production is unencumbered by the demands of consonants. This frees the singer to concentrate on the LMM production of the warm-up vowels, and as a result, they sound wonderful. However, singing a song with words requires the production of *all* phonemes, including the consonants. Because the consonants are produced at a speech speed, the brain turns to "**speech instructions**" in the background processing. But, classical vowel resonance space cannot be maintained with the inter-jection of poorly produced speech consonants. In consequence, the singer loses his or her beautiful sound.

So, what is the LMM? As one yawns, one experiences a relaxation of the muscles at the TMJs that allows the condyles (the top of the mandible that sits in the TMJ) to drop. Try it out: lay your fingers over the TMJ (parallel to your ear) and start a yawn or just drop the jaw. Can you feel how something moves forward and bulges? That is the condyle moving out of the inward curve (mandibular fossa) and gliding forward or translating (a movement of the body in the same direction and at the same rate) into the articular eminence (Figure 3–4).

When one speaks, the condyle rotates mostly in the inward curve (mandibular fossa; hinge motion) with a relatively stable jaw and minimal vertical tongue motion (see the top two skull illustrations in Figure 3–5). For loud speech, there occurs a minor translation along the articular eminence. From this relatively high mandible position, there is not much resonance space available in the oral cavity. Let us test it on ourselves: put your fingers over the TMJ

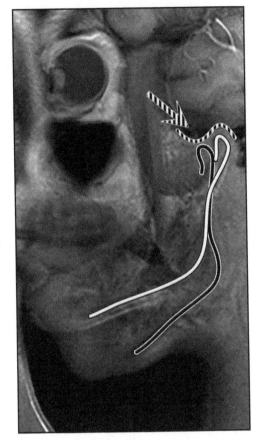

Figure 3–4. A magnetic resonance imaging overlay of the temporomandibular joint of the singer at rest (*white/red*) and performing the low mandible maneuver (LMM) (*black/green*). The LMM condyle position of a sung [ɑ] is indicated by the arrow (Nair et al., 2016).

and feel how little movement there is when you speak. Also, can you feel how little space there is in your oral cavity (move your tongue around) and how easy you can reach the hard palate with the tip of the tongue while barely opening your mouth? This may suffice for the purpose of regular speech. However, a good projected speaking voice in a presentation (with no amplification) or theater requires the same principles as in singing, which is why this book addresses both singers and actors alike.

In singing, the LMM adds an additional maneuver that consists of two interconnected simultaneous actions. Once the condyle reaches the end of the first part of the mouth opening (see previous paragraph), it now starts to translate (a movement of a body in the same direction and at the same rate) over the space between the disc and mandibular fossa (superior joint cavity; see Figure 3–4 and lower two skulls in Figure 3–5).

With that drop, the ramus of the mandible descends, and the **posterior** mandible (the back of the jaw) is lowered. We have measured this drop of the ramus at the mandible angle and have routinely observed a 1- to 1.5-cm drop. With the posterior mandible in a low, relaxed position, more resonance space is established in the oral cavity and the top of the pharyngeal resonance

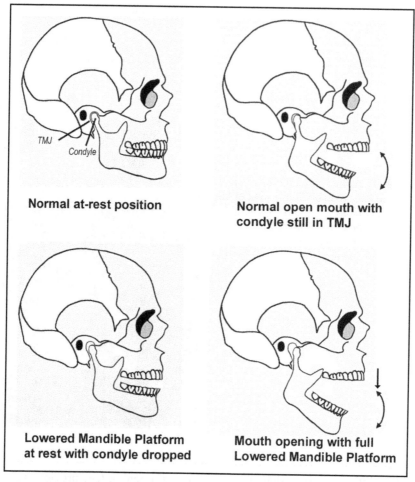

Figure 3–5. Two jaw opening paradigms. The two skulls at the top show the mandible at rest in its normal configuration (left) and the mouth opened (right). The bottom skulls show the low mandible maneuver in operation with the condyle dropped (left) and the resulting increase in mouth opening and oral resonance that results from the maneuver (Nair et al., 2016).

column (see Figure 3–5). Singers tend to raise the soft palate as well, a movement that adds even more space for oral cavity/oropharynx resonance (see Chapter 4).

This increase in oral cavity space, especially at the oropharynx, is why the great pedagogues almost universally call for the yawn as a basis for resonance creation. However, this is not the end of the accumulating benefits for the singer's resonance.

Effects of the Low Mandible Maneuver on the Larynx

The scientific literature has dealt copiously with the effects of the lowered larynx, particularly in classical singing. In Chapter 2, we saw the two groups of the *infrahyoid* (beneath the hyoid) and *suprahyoid* (above the hyoid) muscles and how they are connected to the hyoid bone directly or indirectly.

Most of the explanations of the means by which the larynx is lowered focus on the action of the laryngeal *depressor* muscles (Figure 3–6).

However, as we have seen again and again, one can never single out the interaction of muscle groups, especially in the neck area. We found that the LMM also has a significant role in the *amount* of pharyn-

geal lengthening critical to classical singing resonance. The physical structures of the vocal system are interconnected (see Figures 3–6 and 3–7), so when the back of the jaw (posterior mandible) relaxes downward, the tongue drops with it. In turn, the tongue is connected with the hyoid bone and from there to the larynx.

Subsequently, when this mandible drop occurs, not just the front of the mandible at the chin but also the posterior angle of the

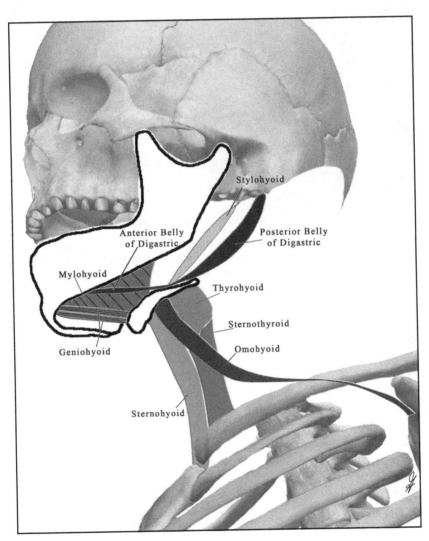

Figure 3–6. Infra- and suprahyoid muscles.

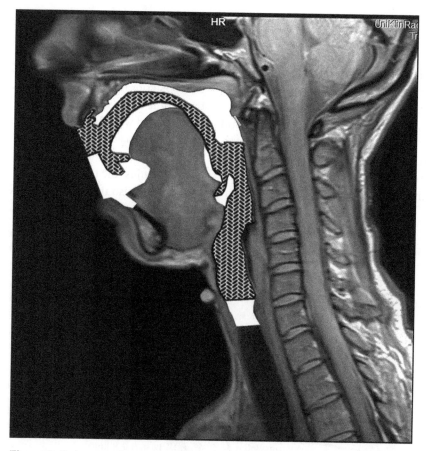

Figure 3–7. Increase in vocal resonance during low mandible maneuver (LMM). The *dark* herringbone area denotes the resonance space available during a non-LMM /i/ vowel. The *white* areas are the spaces that are added during LMM (Nair et al., 2016).

mandible at the back, the larynx drops with it, and the pharynx elongates. The acoustic results of this maneuver are easily seen on a spectrograph in Figure 3–8.

In the LMM research project (Nair et al., 2016), we measured the drop of the larynx both with and without LMM and the differences were significant. We found that a low mandible stance enables the larynx to drop even farther than it can be routinely pulled down by the depressor muscles. In Figure 3–7, one can see the enormous resonance gains through enlargement of space in the oral cavity as well as concomitant resonance pharyngeal area gains because of a significant drop in laryngeal elevation.

In order to achieve the full spectrum of resonance space—as you may have guessed it—we have to look at the suprahyoid (above the hyoid bone) muscles. They are responsible for the elevation of the larynx, and in comparison to the rather similarly formed infrahyoid (below the hyoid bone) muscles, the shape of the suprahyoid muscles is quite different.

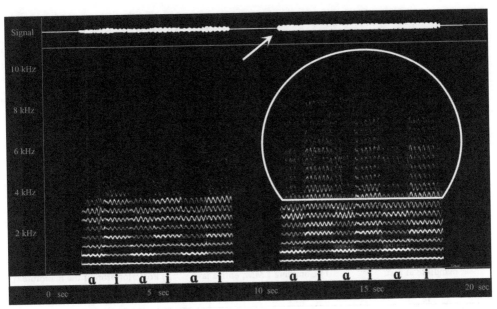

Figure 3–8. Spectrograms of the sung vowels /ɑ/ and /i/; the left shows the acoustic development obtained with an open mouth but not the drop of the posterior mandible. The right images reveal the increases in acoustic development that appear when the whole mandible platform is dropped: more brightness within the harmonics and more upper harmonic (*white/red circle*).

Low Mandible Maneuver Strategies and Posture

Remember the jaw joints (TMJ) just in front of the ears, where the jawbone meets the skull, and the cartilage disc between these two bones, which helps the jaw move smoothly (see earlier). Within the physiological process of the TMJ, there are two strategies that can be applied (Figure 3–9):

▪ the drop of the entire jaw platform; and
▪ the drop of the posterior part of the mandible.

Both strategies enhance the first harmonics, enhance the singer's formant (F_s), and increase the intensity, all of which are the fundamentals we need for good projection in classical singing. However, their application is dependent on the expressive elements of the music at hand, or sometimes even the conductor. For instance, the drop of the entire mandible shows a greater enhancement. Thus, passages that demand greater dynamics, have a large and "thick" orchestration, or need to be sung in a hall/space with acoustical deficiencies, might require an entire mandible drop in order to project appropriately. The second strategy (dropping the posterior part of the mandible) might be used for a more piano (soft) singing, or *messa di voce*. Although the actual mouth opening may seem minimal, however, the drop of the posterior mandible maintains enough enhancement through the widening, openness, and relaxation of the pharyngeal as well as posterior oral cavity. Hence, the voice still contains sufficient core to carry through and project to the audience.

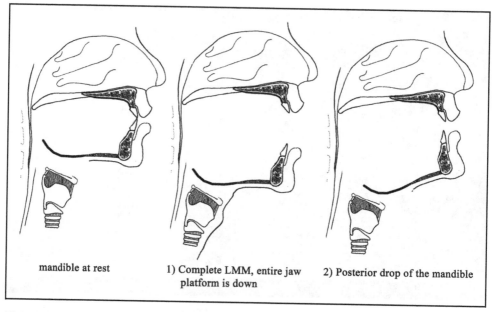

mandible at rest

1) Complete LMM, entire jaw platform is down

2) Posterior drop of the mandible

Figure 3–9. Different mandible strategies: (1) complete low mandible maneuver showing the drop of the entire mandible and (2) Posterior drop of the mandible (Nair et al., 2016).

From an actor's perspective, the first strategy may be used to either increase the dynamic of both vowels and consonants for busy scenes involving crowds or a lot of ambient noise, the need to "shout" the text, or just a poor acoustical environment. The second should be the baseline of our SAS ("say it as a singer") setup, in order to maintain clarity and purity of the overall diction. But, similar to the singers, it helps with the dynamic range, particular for softness, without disappearing or mumbling.

Now, the second strategy may also give a deceptive view of what all the high-ranking singers are actually doing, and that is of great controversy among voice pedagogues and singers. Because of the lack of actual mouth opening, it is believed that one cannot drop and relax the back (posterior) part of the mandible. But as always, the "proof of the pudding lies in the eating." So, try it out yourself.

Temporomandibular Joint— Exercise (Figure 3–10)

Take a pencil and place it in a way so that it is about a quarter of an inch (64 mm) behind your front teeth (like biting on a cigar). Slowly start to move your jaw back and forth, and you will see the pencil tip go up and down with it (depending on the length of your pencil, the tip will move accordingly: up to the level of your eyes and out of sight). Now put your fingers on your TMJ, focus on the condyle, and imagine that it glides forward on a smooth track. (This helps avoid clenching the jaw when initiating the move or focusing on moving the chin up and forward.) You will feel again—as we already experienced earlier—how the condyle bulges and translates forward. You may support that thought with letting go/elongating the big masseter muscle (in your cheeks at the corner of the

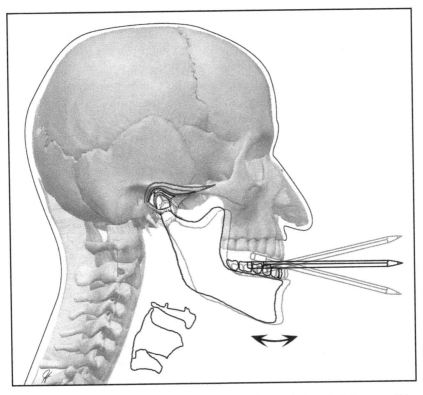

Figure 3–10. Exercise for the drop of the back (posterior) part of the mandible.

jaw) as well as starting to massage around your temporal and cheekbone. In addition, with the acquired knowledge of the infrahyoid muscles (the muscles between the jaw/skull and hyoid bone), support the forward movement by imagining how these muscles elongate/widen and how the mylohyoid, in particular, turns into a downward relaxed wide carpet (it almost turns into a gobbler under a chin). Can you feel how your larynx drops, the pharynx and posterior oral cavity elongates/opens up while still holding your pencil with your teeth? You may even trigger a yawn because of that relaxation (a good sign). Finally, sing on a comfortable pitch, and slowly make the movement so you can feel the difference in singing (record it also so you can listen to the difference in resonance of the sung tone).

This exercise not only shows you that, even though the mouth itself may not be wide open, one can still drop/open up the back (posterior) part of the mandible and subsequently sing with a nice open and resonant tone. It is also a wonderful exercise that will help relax the chewing muscles (temporalis, masseter, etc.). A lot of times they spasm because of teeth grinding, stress, anxiety, tiredness, and emotional upset, to name a few. If that happens, it causes the disc to become displaced, leading to a clicking when opening the mouth (the disc is in the way or tries to get back into place) or an inflamed painful joint. Starting a warm-up routine with this exercise really gets everything loose and ready.

Continuing in the spirit of relaxation let us add another exercise for muscles that are prone to spasm because of poor posture, anxiety, stress, emotional upset, and so forth: the short neck muscles (see Chapter 2). The following little exercise will help relax the muscles with a myofascial release of the short neck muscles (suboccipital muscles), so we are not blocking the relaxed movement we already established in the TMJ and mandible.

Neck Muscle (Suboccipital Muscles)—Exercise (Figure 3–11)

Before we start the following exercise, you need to get two tennis balls to roll back and forth on. To make this easier, you can either put the balls into a sock, or duct tape them so they stay together and, as you will see, roll along each side of your spine without slipping away. Now, you need to lay down on your back (supine), tuck your feet in at a 90° angle (to align your lumbar curve with the floor), and put the balls underneath your neck right where the base of the skull is. Put your hands on the side of the balls to keep them in place and start tucking your chin, rolling back and forth on the

balls. To make that process of antagonism as easy and natural as possible, find out which focus helps you not to force the movement. For instance, when you move the chin up, connect that movement by focusing either (a) on the contraction of the short neck muscle so the front side (anterior) of the neck (supra- and infrahyoid muscles, larynx) relaxes and expands/widens naturally or (b) on the expansion/relaxation of the front so the short neck muscles contract naturally. That way we keep the joint of skull and spine (atlas and axis) free while massaging the fasciae of the muscles surrounding them. Repeat the rolling about 10 to 15 times and then move the position of the balls to the outside, away from the spine so one ball will be on the spine and the other on the side of the neck. Again, roll for 10 to 15 times and repeat on the opposite side. That way we cover the entire area along the bottom of the skull. Also, make sure the rolls are nice and easy and the movements are slow, so we have a myofascial release in the area (possibly a bit painful because of the tension) and no unintentional tightening.

Do you notice a release within the short neck muscles, the mandible, shoulders, and/

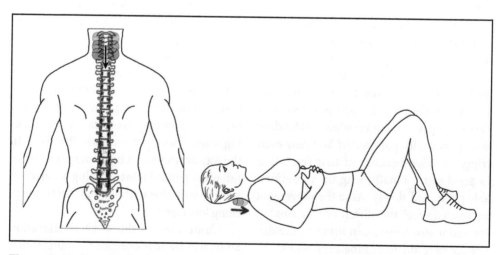

Figure 3–11. Exercise for the short neck muscles (suboccipital muscles).

or entire back/upper body? If not, do not worry; keep working at it, and no matter what exercise you do, I suggest you do not just focus on the execution of the exercise itself. Once you are clear on how to do it, observe the effect and/or sensation at the very spot of the exercise as well as how it may spread and/or affect other parts of your body. After all, everything is connected within our body, so just observe and enjoy any evolving sensations.

Effect of the Low Mandible Maneuver on the Tongue

So far, we explored the entire structure of the mandible and neck in order to accomplish the five points, reviewed at the beginning, that a maximum resonance creation depends on: open mouth and oral cavity, elongated pharynx, relaxation of muscles at and around the TMJ for the LMM, lower larynx. Though – yes you guessed it, the LMM has not only an effect on the larynx but, since everything is connected, on the tongue as well.

The tongue is an incredible, mobile structure and one of the most malleable articulators. Later in this book, we see how it can form itself acrobatically into the most remarkable shapes. This is not only true for vowels but for what is at the core of this book—consonants. As singers, we need to ensure intelligibility while maintaining the most resonant sound. Hence, the slightest change of the shape of the tongue affects not only the resulting phoneme but its acousti-

cal outcome (intensity) and timbre as well. The same is true for actors, even if it is not to the full extent as for singers.

In Chapter 2, we saw the complexity of the intrinsic (originate and insert within the tongue) and extrinsic (linked to surrounding bones and tissue) tongue muscles and how they enable the tongue to extend and retract at the same time. Our body's muscular system comprises different types of muscle tissue. In general, locomotion, maintenance of posture, and other muscular activities depend on the interaction of muscles with a system of skeletal support. The nervous system[1] sends a signal to the muscle to contract, and the bone follows, giving support to the contracting muscles starting the action (agonist) as well as the relaxing muscles opposing the action (antagonist).[2] In addition, we need to keep in mind that no matter if the muscle contracts or expands, it will change in length and/or size and stay in a more or less restricted area.

The tongue, on the other hand, is an organ that is considered a muscular-hydrostat (Kier & Smith, 1985). Earlier, we mentioned that skeletal muscles get their support from the bone. However, the tongue is composed *entirely of muscles* and *does not change its volume*. The former means that the musculature itself both creates movement and provides skeletal support for that movement. The latter, on the other hand, is of particular interest because it is the most important biomechanical feature of a muscular-hydrostat: *the volume of the structure is constant*. This means that the tongue muscles are responsible for both *moving* and *shaping* the tongue, making it one of

---

[1]Our brain is the command center of our body; in order to understand how signals are sent out when you want to move, one needs to know more about the central nervous system and brain. For better insight on the matter, you can find a succinct and nontechnical overview of the central and peripheral nervous system in the book *Articulatory Phonetics* (2013), by Gick, Wilson, and Derrick.
[2]The bone also amplifies the forces that come with it (e.g., speed or displacement of muscular activity).

the most flexible parts of our body. To help you visualize this fascinating feature, imagine a water balloon in your hands: no matter how you squeeze, dent, or pinch it, only the shape and/or surface will change, while the volume/size will always stay the same. Thus, compression in one location means expansion in another (Kier & Smith, 1985; Smith & Kier, 1989).

With the entire or the posterior mandible dropped, the singer's tongue is no longer as proximate to the palate as it is in everyday speech. This dictates that classical singers must significantly rehabituate the use of the tongue—it must simultaneously be far more active on the vertical plane in order to both produce clear diction and maintain the increased resonance created by the low mandible. Because everyday speech is so automatic for the singer, the process of learning this new tongue-shape paradigm is necessarily a lengthy one that routinely takes years to accomplish. And, considering the second strategy of the LMM as a baseline of our SAS setup, the same is true for actors. And as mentioned earlier, no matter how small or large the movement we make with this muscular organ, it is always accompanied by deformation of the entire tongue. Do you begin to see the challenges and why we often feel like we have a "knot" in our tongue?

Now that the LMM concept has been introduced to you, it is time to show its ramifications for tongue shapes.

In Figure 3–12, magnetic resonance imaging clearly shows the substantial differences in the actual tongue shape and position for the spoken and sung vowels as well as the two different strategies of LMM

indicated by the checker striped/yellow line. In addition, they demonstrate its effect on the increase of vocal resonance space. The singing profile for the back vowel /ɑ/ shows an increase in both the posterior resonance space (adding to the oropharynx, mouth, and space above larynx) as well as the anterior space increase in the front of the mouth (see also Figure 3–7). Also note that the apex (tip) of the tongue profile is shifted back in the mouth, and the wave line of the tongue surface is more pronounced. For the /i/, again, there is an increase in both the oropharyngeal and the front of oral cavity space. The apex of the tongue is not only shifted back but also retracted within the elongated tongue.

Congratulations. You made it through the fascinatingly complex anatomical structures of the (for our purpose) most important parts of the body. It may seem daunting at first to have to know all of this. That is why I am suggesting you do not even think that way. You can always come back to these chapters and look up the names and locations of the muscles. Just start by looking at the muscle concept first, what the function of the muscle is and how the muscles are connected to each other. I am sure that after a while, you may subconsciously start to even remember the particular names. Although we like to think of ourselves as multitaskers, we are only able to focus on one thing at a time. So, give yourself the time to get familiar with the concept by focusing on one puzzle piece at a time, and I am sure you will soon be able to gradually put all of the pieces together. With that spirit, let us move on to the next piece of the puzzle.

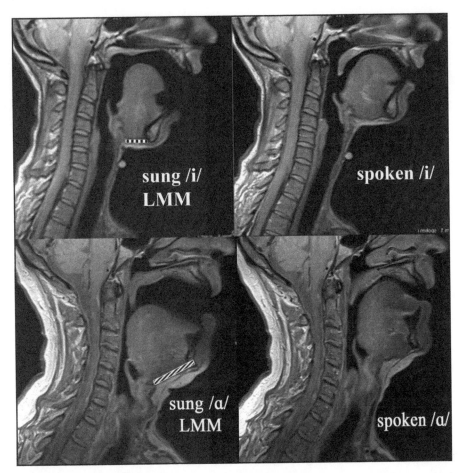

Figure 3–12. Top right image, spoken /i/, and the left image, sung /i/ with full classical resonance. Note the drop of the mandible and the larynx. Bottom images show spoken /ɑ/ (*right*) and sung /ɑ/ (*left*) with full classical resonance. Also note the different angles following the low mandible maneuver (*checker striped/yellow line*) (Nair et al., 2016).

References

Gick, B., Wilson, I., & Derrick, D. (2013) *Articulatory phonetics*. West Sussex, UK. Wiley-Blackwell

Howard, D. M., & Murphy, D. T. (2008). *Voice science, acoustics and recording*. San Diego, CA: Plural Publishing.

Kier, W. M., & Smith, K. K. (1985). Tongues, tentacles and trunks: The biomechanics of movement in muscular-hydrostats. *Zoological Journal of the Linnean Society, 83,* 307–324.

Nair, A., Nair, G., & Reishofer, G. (2016). The low mandible maneuver and its resonential implications for elite singers. *Journal of Voice, 30,* 128.e13–128.e32.

Sataloff, R. T. (2005). *Professional voice: The science and art of clinical care* (3rd ed.). San Diego, CA: Plural Publishing.

Smith, K. K., & Kier, W. M. (1989). Trunks, tongues, and tentacles: Moving with skeletons of muscle. *American Scientist, 77,* 28–35.

4 Watch Your Tongue

First of all, "no worries." In this chapter, I am not asking you to be careful of what you are actually saying. Rather, let me ask you: have you ever watched and/or consciously paid attention to your tongue when you talk or eat? Chances are that the answer is likely to be "no," which is not that surprising. Even within our automated speech template, oral sensory awareness and perception of the precise position of our tongue are often a challenging task. Let's face it, who ever thought about how or where to put the tongue for the vowel /e/ or the consonant /r/, unless there has been some sort of phonological or articulatory disorder in childhood—or you had a good voice teacher. This is compounded by the relative lack of tongue proprioceptors (nerve endings that transfer information concerning position and movement in the body to the brain) and the complexity of tongue muscles (see Chapter 2). Thus, to attain deliberate control requires slow development of precise motor sensory skills of tongue movements.

In Chapter 2 we introduced the effect of the low mandible maneuver (LMM) on the tongue. With the body of the entire tongue (average 9 cm[1]) occupying the majority of the oropharyngeal cavity (mouth and throat) and the comparison of spoken and sung front vowels, those elaborate changes are even more obvious (see Chapter 3, Figure 3–10). So, the question arises: how can we deliberately maneuver the tongue into such acrobatic shapes? Part II of this book answers that question in detail for every consonant. In the next chapters though, we continue to look deeper into the building blocks of spoken language and the various tongue shapes of vowels and consonants. But first, let us start by gaining more awareness, flexibility, and control through some tongue exercises that are also very useful as a warm-up regimen.

In previous chapters, we learned about the jaw joint (temporomandibular joint, or TMJ) and used exercises to learn how to execute the two different strategies of the LMM and relax the chewing muscles. But before we started with the exercise, we looked at the anatomy and physiology of the area concerned, so we could put our focus on it during the exercise and create awareness. As in sports and other physical activities, we need to train our body, or certain parts of it, to move in particularly efficient ways. It is what Ericsson calls "deliberate practice" and "mental representation."[2] However, in order to habituate neuromuscular behavior (e.g., singing, speaking), one must also have an accurate knowledge of the result (KR) (Maas et al., 2008; Verdolini &

---

[1]Sanders et al. (2013).
[2]Ericsson and Pool (2016).

Krebs, 1999). Broadly speaking, one needs to know how to execute the skill (deliberate practice) within a pool of knowledge concerning the area at hand, as well as have a clear idea of the aimed outcome (mental representation).

But how can we increase our oral sensory awareness? Learning how to consciously maneuver our tongue in singing or speaking is similar to how we as babies started to acquire language or sensory experiences (i.e., touch). Thus, we need to start with baby steps to acquire the control necessary for vowels and consonants. Speech-language pathologists use forms of oral sensory-motor treatment, such as oral placement therapy (OPT) and phonetic placement therapy (PPT),[3] to help clients with speech and swallowing disorders. Both therapies use techniques such as touch, movement, and tools (like your own hands) to help increase the oral sensory awareness and sustained muscle activity of the tongue, lips, and jaw.

However, it seems as though when we attempt an involuntary or unconsciously habituated movement, like breathing or moving the tongue, it often feels foreign or even impossible to execute it, as if we have forgotten how to do it. To overcome this obstacle, let us work through some exercises to increase awareness, flexibility, and control that have experientially been proven helpful in learning to deliberately maneuver the tongue. At first, it is helpful to use a mirror or the reverse camera of your smartphone as a guide and for better control. However, before we continue, a disclaimer is in order. Although the following exercises will not harm the tongue, the participant might look a bit silly. For this, I will not take any responsibility and will only say, "Have fun with it!"

Tongue Warm-Up and Strengthening Exercises

We start with exercises that can be used both as a warm-up as well as to strengthen the tongue.

- **Rest your tongue** on the roof of the mouth and bite down so that your back teeth are together, lips closed. Hold for 30 sec and then try to swallow (*note:* keep the contact with the roof of the mouth while you swallow).
- **Monkey face:** put your tongue over the front teeth, under your upper lips, hold for 10 sec and then relax (repeat 10 times); hold your tongue against your lower lip, hold for 10 sec (repeat 10 times).
- Put the **tip of the tongue** behind your upper teeth (alveolar ridge), hold it, and then, while keeping the contact, start to open and close your jaw.
- **Tongue pull:** take a strip from a paper towel so you do not slip when you grab your tongue tip (apex):
  1. Gently pull out (straight) your tongue, hold for 1 min (build up to 5 min).
  2. Gently pull to the right, hold, and then to the left, hold.
  3. Gently pull the tongue up and then down and hold on each.
- **Tongue push:** Take a spoon, popsicle, or the like and push your tongue against it for 10 sec.
- **Tongue push-up:** push your tongue up against a spoon or popsicle 10 times (*note:* keep the jaw open, relaxed, and not moving with the tongue).
- **Chewing on the tongue:** imagine your tongue being a nice big ball of gum that you twist a little while you are chewing

---

[3]"Phonetic placement therapy" was the term used before Sara Rosenfeld-Johnson coined the term "oral placement therapy."

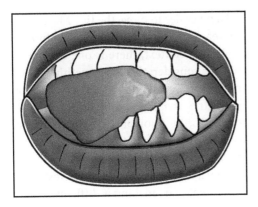

Figure 4–1. Chewing on the gum.

it between your teeth (Figure 4–1). Try to chew every part of the tongue by moving it between all your teeth, front to back (canines, incisors, premolars, and molars). Should you feel some pain at first, start gently and slowly increase the intensity of your bite.

Exercise 2

Next, start by moving the tip of the tongue around the mouth, drawing big circles on the palate from the outside to the inside and back out, changing the direction (Figure 4–2). Take note of all the surface irregularities, the sensation within the tip of the tongue, and how your entire tongue behaves in order to complete the task. Do the sensations within the tongue tip change from more noticeable to less? Is it easy for you to guide the tip? Do you feel any resistance in the tongue root and/or middle of the tongue surface when you want to move in a particular direction? If there is any tension building up, reset and start over. This time, try to maintain the contact of the tip of the tongue to the palate without force or push from the back of the tongue and imagine the center of the tongue to be like an elastic, almost fluid silicon.

Let us continue our "oral cleansing" by moving the tip behind our lips and start with small circles (four to five rounds, building up to 15). Continue to expand the movement all over the entire mouth, going around the outside of the upper and lower teeth, as if cleaning them, and try, if you can, to get around the lower back teeth and around the floor of the mouth (which

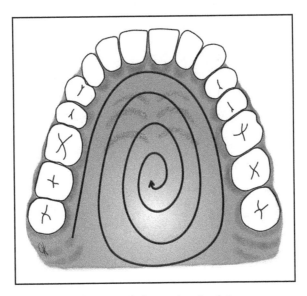

Figure 4–2. Tongue circles on hard palate.

houses a series of saliva gland ducts). Again, any noticeable blockages within the tongue along the way?

Sometimes, the root of the tongue can get stiff through trying to move around. Why? Looking at Figure 4–3, the tongue, or blade of the tongue, is the portion that extends from the tip of your tongue and is the part of the tongue that lies directly under the arch of the hard palate and upper front teeth (alveolar ridge) when the tongue is at rest in a closed mouth (Ladefoged & Maddieson, 1996). It is rather small in proportion when compared to the rest, not directly attached to the bottom of the mouth, and we can actually stick it out. Now, it is not uncommon for people to try to move the tip with pushes from the big genioglossus (GG) muscle (see Figure 4–3). Subsequently, the tip may curl a bit, but the rest of the tongue becomes somewhat blocked, trying to "muscle" its way around. Should you have the sensation of a blockage while trying to maneuver your tongue tip through the mouth, imagine letting go/releasing that big fan-like muscle (genioglossus). Does it

feel a bit easier to move the tip? Maybe you can reach even further back than before?

In this context, there is one important thing to consider: there is something called tongue-tie, or ankyloglossia. This occurs when the strip of skin connecting the tongue to the floor of the mouth (lingual frenulum) is shorter than usual. Some of those who have it do not seem to be bothered by it. Others may experience restricted movement (e.g., making it difficult to stick their tongue out of their mouth). Should you happen to be limited in your movements because of a tongue-tie (minor or major), I would encourage you to work on relaxing and stretching the tongue because the compensation of limited mobility can often result in stiffening of the tongue root, which, in turn, puts strain on the throat.

Exercise 3

The next exercise is a good stretch of the tongue. As you know, the tongue is solely composed of muscles, and these muscles

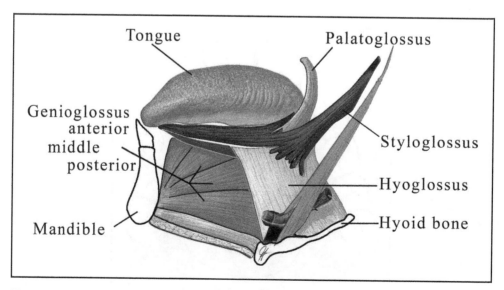

Figure 4–3. Extrinsic tongue muscles.

need to be stretched in the same way as athletes stretch their leg muscles. However, before we start with an exercise, let us stretch the tongue manually. Though I have to warn you, this will most likely not feel very pleasant or may even hurt a little, particularly if you have never done anything like it. Nevertheless, this should be—as with any massage, trigger points, and so on—a "good pain" (pain that ends immediately after you stop the activity), where you gently work your way through it and almost simultaneously start to notice the gradual relaxation following it, particularly after you are done. In general, exercises stretch and cause small tears in muscles (that includes

the vocal fold when singing) that, in turn, stimulate them to grow bigger and stronger. Unless you do it excessively, the soreness will subside within a day or so and not impede your ability to perform normal daily activities or keep you from moving your tongue.

With those "cheerful" perspectives, let us start: with your index finger and thumb, form a "c" (Figure 4–4) and put a strip of paper towel along the inside, so you have an easier time grabbing your tongue and do not slip. To avoid any gagging or other rather unpleasant sensations, start to slowly move your fingers into your mouth by moving along the bottom teeth, going deep down to the bottom of the tongue. Do not rush

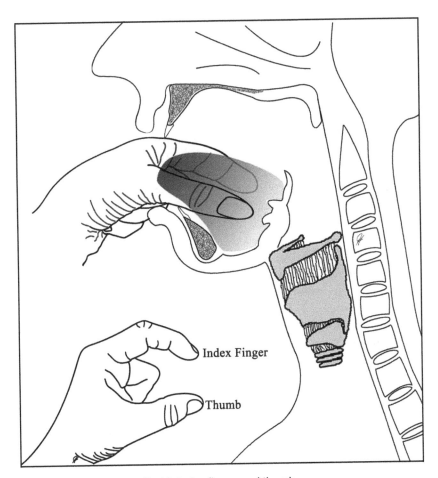

Index Finger

Thumb

Figure 4–4. Tongue-pull with index finger and thumb.

it, and get used to the "foreign" object in your mouth. Once you reached as far back as possible, begin squeezing the root. Again, try to find a bearable level of pain, since this will likely hurt. Continue for a minute and then release. Repeat a few times or keep at it as long as you can (start with three times first and build up repetitions and time).

Next, grab the root of the tongue, and gently pull the tongue straight outward and feel the stretch within the tongue itself as well as in the surroundings (e.g., the palatoglossus [the side walls running down from the uvula into the tongue] and down to the larynx). Observe what happens when you pull. For example, does the larynx move up as well? Do you feel tension in the larynx? You may even want to take the other hand and gently move the larynx downward in the opposite direction. This will not only help you stretch both tongue and laryngeal muscles but also help in the discernment of whether there is a buildup of tension and how to possibly let go through relaxation. And, let us not forget the TMJ (see Chapter 2) that may also be in need of some relaxation.

As stated earlier, to create independence between the phonatory (larynx) and articulatory (in this case primarily the tongue, but also the TMJ), we have to start slowly and gently. Start the exercise with two to three repetitions and gradually increase them. Also, after each massage and/or pull, notice any change in the tongue, TMJ, neck, or the entire vocal tract for that matter. Did the level of awareness of the tongue in your oral (mouth) and pharyngeal cavity (throat) increase? Does the tongue feel more relaxed, maybe even more voluminous (after all, the tongue occupies more than half of the vocal tract, see Chapter 2)? If so, great. If not, do not worry, to build a motor sensory connection is a slow and complex process. Also, do not worry if there is an increase of your saliva production. The movement of the tongue massages the small glands directly underneath the tongue that squeeze out saliva. So, the next time you encounter a dry mouth, either do this exercise or simply bite the edges of your tongue (very helpful before or during a performance).

Exercise 4

Let us continue with our next exercise. Roll your tongue tip up to the hard palate and then see how far back your tongue is able to go (Figure 4–5). Hold your tongue back until it feels too uncomfortable. Repeat the exercise three to four times and pay attention to the root of the tongue. Is it relaxed enough that the tip can move freely and maybe even farther back? Were you able to reach the soft palate or even your uvula this time? No worries, if not; what is important is working step by step to stretch it and increase flexibility.

Of course, we should balance out the movement. Start by sticking out your tongue down to your chin, while opening your jaw by relaxing the muscles around the jaw joint (TMJ) like a snake or lizard. Make sure that your throat is relaxed, not tense, because it also wants to push out the tongue. Imagine it as if you are uncoupling your tongue from your larynx, moving them diagonally in opposite directions. Also, by looking at Figure 4–3, imagine relaxing the following muscles: genioglossus, hyoglossus, and palatoglossus. Notice which relaxation was most helpful to you in only moving out the surface of the tongue (tongue blade). Return to the starting position, and repeat the exercise three to four times.

Exercise 5

Next, open your jaw and anchor your tongue tip behind your lower teeth, then roll the

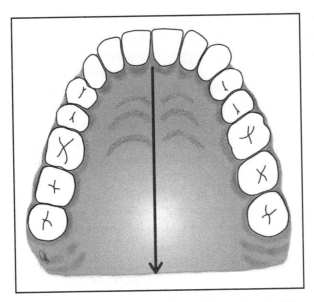

Figure 4–5. Tongue moves straight back on hard palate.

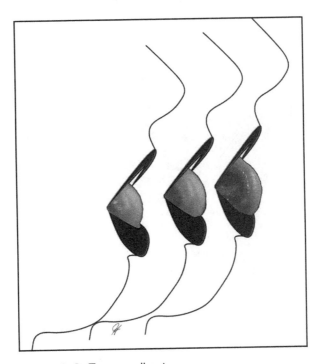

Figure 4–6. Tongue roll-out.

back of your tongue forward and out of your mouth (Figure 4–6). Again, pay attention to your larynx, keeping it relaxed while creating more space in the back of your mouth.

Besides stretching and increasing tongue awareness, our goal is to independently move and hold the tongue, jaw, and larynx without any tension. This will enable us to use our filter (articulators, particularly the tongue and jaw) without interfering with the relaxed state of the source (the larynx) (see Chapter 5).

Before we continue, it is worth refreshing your memory of the tongue muscles (see Chapter 2, Figures 2–7 and 2–8). Remember the intrinsic tongue muscles that I described as being layered like a peanut butter and jelly sandwich (Figure 4–7)? The superior and inferior longitudinal muscles are like two bread slices, and the transversalis and verticalis muscles are the peanut butter and jelly. Let us see how to develop some awareness of the transversalis (T) and verticalis (V) muscles.

Keep your lips together and stick out your tongue. Now change the shape from flat to round and repeat it a couple of times (Figure 4–8). Our peanut butter and jelly

(transversalis, narrows/elongates; verticalis, flattens/broadens) are responsible for narrowing/elongating and flattening/broadening the tongue. If your tongue wants to get into a "u" shape, then your genioglossus (big fan-shaped muscle on the tongue bottom) most likely depresses the midline instead of protruding it (like giving support upward). You may use your front teeth—that hold your tongue between them—as feedback, where the tongue acts like an automobile jack, expanding in the center to push them apart.

Exercise 6

The next exercise is going to be interesting and, experientially, has been shown to be very beneficial and revealing of one's

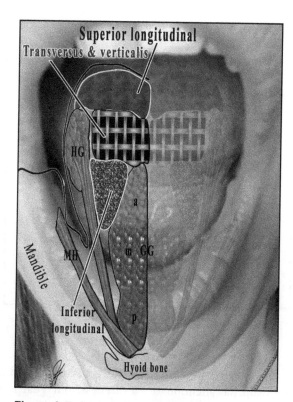

Figure 4–7. Intrinsic tongue muscles.

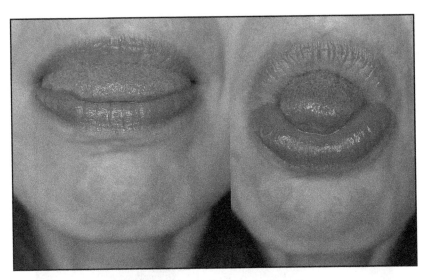

Figure 4–8. Transversalis and verticalis muscles in action.

tongue behavior in general. First, we need a "tongue depressor." This might be a flat, thin, wooden blade, smoothed and rounded at both ends, similar to that which is used by doctors to examine your mouth and throat, or maybe even a wooden spoon or stick, to help feel and guide your tongue. So, let us get started: the inferior (I) and superior longitudinal (SL) muscles (see Figure 4–7) are responsible for shortening the tongue and curling the tip (apex). Imagine the blade of the tongue (the one you can stick out) laying on a rail track where the inferior longitudinal muscles are your two tracks and the surface of the tongue (superior muscles) is a lid that slides on them (see Figure 4–8). Using the tongue depressor, place it on the front part of your tongue (blade) to establish contact, and then start moving the tongue (Figure 4–9). Does it feel difficult to move the tongue? Do you sense tension and/or blockages, particularly in the tongue root, because you stabilized the tip?

It is interesting that eliminating the movement of the tongue tip results in a paresis of the rest of the tongue. Similarly, it shows that we lock-in other muscles so

we can move the tip. The following example illustrates the principle in a broader sense. Imagine turning your nose in small movements (half an inch) to the left and then to the right, like drawing a short line with your nose by wiggling continuously "no." Do you have a hard time moving only your head without your entire body—starting with the shoulders trying to turn with it also? If so, this is because we subconsciously think that we need to lock-in all of our muscles just to accomplish a tiny little task such as the wiggling of our nose. More often than not, we are locking our joints, muscles, and fasciae when trying to execute a movement of a particular body part. In the same context, as we already touched on in Chapter 2 (agonist–antagonist), the skull has a joint in the first two vertebrae (atlas and axis) connected through ligaments and muscles. Locking them will result in rigidity of the entire neck and spine, thus moving the entire body when only the head should move.

Coming back to our tongue, just as we ideally seek independence between the head and spine, we now want independence within the tongue: the base/root of

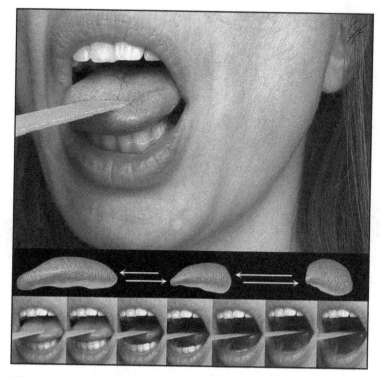

Figure 4–9. Contraction and expansion of inferior and superior longitudinal muscles using a tongue depressor for guidance.

the tongue and tongue blade. Let us see if we can help free up our tongue with the help of touch and visual aids. Start again by putting the tongue depressor on the front of the tongue and look at Figure 4–2. Drop the jaw in a relaxed manner and imagine the back sides of the tongue (hyoglossus) relaxing with it. Slowly start retracting only your tongue blade (see Figure 4–9), and envision the genioglossus and hyoglossus as being relaxed, almost unperturbed by the "lid" sliding like a curved back and down (into your pharynx) movement. If you find yourself struggling to get it to a similar outcome as in Figure 4–9, it is likely that you are trying to curl the tip up and downward in order to get the tongue back, while flexing/locking the genioglossus and its neighbors. Another way to get more flexibility is to gently bite on the edges of your tongue, like a massage, before you repeat the exercise. Then, try it again and release the tension in these edges, imagining the hyoglossus to be like reins pulling back the tongue. Our goal is to focus on shortening the tongue only and leaving the tip in a "neutral" position.

Unfortunately, we do not see a lot of the genioglossus (GG) when looking into the mirror. However, there is enough visible for us to learn and start a motor sensory connection and increase the awareness with another exercise. Figure 4–10A shows the GG in a depressed state. You can see that the contours of wings—looking similar to the vocal folds during breathing—are more pronounced, while with a protruded GG they move forward and almost disappear (Figure 4–10B).

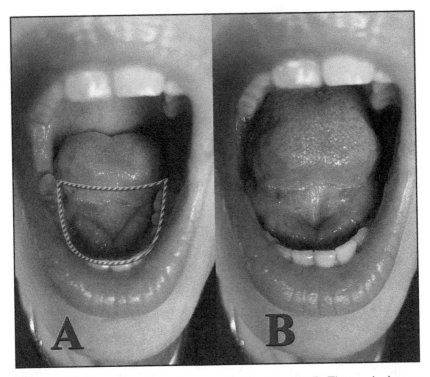

Figure 4–10. A. The genioglossus in depressed state. **B.** The genioglossus protruded.

When doing this exercise, keep the upper body of the tongue retracted and feel the difference in your pharynx. The challenge is to perform the movement of the GG independent of the larynx (i.e., not initiating the push from the larynx in order to avoid it raising and tensing). Place the tops of two fingers underneath the chin and feel the push from the GG against your fingers. If you do not feel anything, the push is most likely initiated by the larynx.

Whereas the previous exercise focused on upward movements for front vowels, such as /e/ (s<u>ay</u>), movements in the opposite direction—depressing the GG, for vowels such as /æ/ (th<u>a</u>t) and /ɑ/ (l<u>a</u>w), as well as for central and back vowels (see Chapter 6)—can be equally challenging. However, the results can be seen and monitored more eas-

ily in the mirror (Figure 4–11A). Open and relax your jaw, then lay down your tongue on the floor of the mouth. Now use the depressing motion from the previouse exercise to create a groove in the tongue (Figure 4–11B). Again, use your fingers under your chin to help direct the depression of the GG muscle vertically down and not backward. Should you have a hard time keeping your tongue relaxed, or should your tip tend to move around a lot, take your tongue depressor to calm down the movement.

I hope that this oral-motor workout has not only relaxed and loosened your tongue overall but also given you more flexibility in, and awareness of its movement. The more malleable the tongue becomes in manipulating the shapes of its different parts, the more flexibility and control we have to

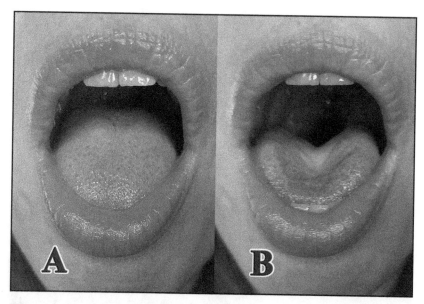

Figure 4–11. A. Neutral tongue shape. **B.** Tongue with the genioglossus depressed.

influence the dimensions and proportion of our metaphorical two-room/hallway (see Chapter 5). As a result, this will not only help us to shape and place the proper phonemes for intelligibility and resonance but also enable us to change the timbre (tone color) for emotional content. So, let us look next at the various acrobatics and shapes the tongue can perform and form.

References

Ericsson, K. A., & Pool, R. (2016). *Peak: The secrets from the new science of expertise.* Boston, MA: Houghton Mifflin Harcourt.

Ladefoged, P., & Maddieson, I. (1996). *The sounds of the world's languages.* Malden, MA: Blackwell Publishers.

Maas, E., Robin, D. A., Austermann Hula, S. N., Freedman, S. E., Wulf G., Ballard, K. J., & Schmidt, R. A. (2008). Principles of motor learning in treatment of motor speech disorders. *American Journal of Speech-Language Pathology, 17,* 277–298.

Sanders, I., Mu, L., Amirali, A., Su, H., & Sobotka, S. (2013). The human tongue slows down to speak: Muscle fibers of the human tongue. *Anatomical Record* (Hoboken), *296*(10), 1615–1627.

Verdolini, K., & Krebs, D. (1999). Some considerations on the science of special challenges in voice training. In G. Nair (Ed.), *Voice tradition and technology: A state-of-the-art studio* (pp. 227–239). San Diego, CA: Singular Publishing.

5 The Building Blocks of Language and Biofeedback From Ultrasound

Before launching our study of singing languages, some definitions are necessary. Phonetics is the study of speech sounds, their articulations, acoustics properties, as well as perception. For singers and actors, the approach of language needs to be like that of a phonetician. This is especially true working with languages whose letters and combinations of letters require phonemes that are different from those of our own native language or dialect.

All languages consist of strings of **phonemes**. A phoneme is a single language sound, regardless of how it is produced by the human voice. For instance, the word *phoneme* is constructed out of the following language sounds:

$$/fo^unim/$$

This example has been written in the **International Phonetic Alphabet** (IPA), an alphabet that contains most of the sounds needed to transliterate most of the world's languages. Sometimes we are unaware of the sounds of our own language and confuse the letters of the alphabet with the sound of the language. In this example, note that the phonemes (each individual letter) do not follow the way the word is spelled but rather the way it *sounds*. *Note:* the author superscripts the secondary vowel of diphthongs in IPA in order to aid in identifying which vowel to sustain while singing multiple notes occurring on the same syllable.

In our example, the written "ph" is one of the 11 different ways /f/ can be written in English. When we look again at our example, the written "ph" is one of the different ways /f/ can be written (Table 5–1).

The long English "o" is actually a **diphthong**, a combination of two adjacent vowel sounds, one executed longer than the other ($/o^u/$).

Finishing with our example, the /i/ is the symbol for the English long ee sound. Notice that there is no "e" after the /m/. In English, many words feature a silent "e," most commonly at the end of a word. However, it was pronounced before historical

Table 5–1. A Selection of the Different Ways /f/ Can Be Written in English

Spelling	Word	International Phonetic Alphabet
ph	<u>ph</u>oneme	fo^{u}nim
f	<u>f</u>ine	fʌ^{i}n
ff	stu<u>ff</u>	stʌf
gh	enou<u>gh</u>	ɪnʌf

55

sound changes, such as the Great Vowel Shift, occurred.

The beauty of IPA is that the symbol /i/ stands for that phoneme no matter what language we are working with (Table 5–2).

Anyone who has their first encounter with IPA is often afraid of having to learn so many different symbols. However, to help ease that fear, the map *The Familiar IPA* by Garyth Nair (2007) will show that you probably know much more of the IPA than you think (Figure 5–1).

Follow the boxes from the inside out, starting with the gray box. The sounds that these letters stand for in those languages are the same for IPA. The IPA letters in the next box, as the title implies, stand for the same phonemes as they do in English. Moving to the outer box, we can see new symbols. However, they are connected to certain phonemes in the two inner boxes because they all have a relationship in shape as well as sound. So, the only symbols one has to really learn in order to transliterate German, French, and Italian are the little boxes on the bottom.

We utilize the IPA extensively throughout this book because a working knowledge of it makes mastering languages used in singing and acting so much easier.

Now, say the word to yourself in slow motion, and you will hear the constituent phonemes we just dissected in the word *phoneme*—/fo^{u}nim/.

Classification of Sounds

There are two types of phonemes: **vowels** and **consonants**.

The definition of the word *vowel* usually focuses on statements such as *a language sound that is produced with an open vocal tract*.

To get a sense of this definition, "say it as a singer" (SAS) or sing several vowels, /i/ /æ/ /ɑ/ and /u/ while looking at the requisite sagittal (side) images of the tongue as shown in Figure 5–2. In this series of vowels, the resonance space (air), white space, is continuous from where it begins in the pharynx at the right to the opening at the lips on the left.

Open Vocal Tract

Reverting to Figure 5–2, you will notice that the tongue (darker gray) is shaped differently for each of these four vowels. Each shape creates, in effect, two "rooms" with the connecting "hallway" (the space above the narrowest channel between tongue and palate). It is the relative shape and size of the two "rooms" that is the acoustic reason that each of these phonemes sound as they do. Because of the hallway above the tongue, the vocal tract is still considered open. Hence, vowels are produced by an open vocal tract that is more or less unobstructed. The only contact being made by the tongue—though more so in speech than in singing—is with the upper and lower teeth and their corre-

Table 5–2. Examples of the International Phonetic Alphabet (IPA) Symbol /i/ in Various Languages

Language	Word	Word in IPA
English	phoneme	/fo^{u}nim/
French	oui	/^{w}i/
Italian	si	/si/
Russian	пить	/p^{j}it^{j}/
German	siehe	/ziə/

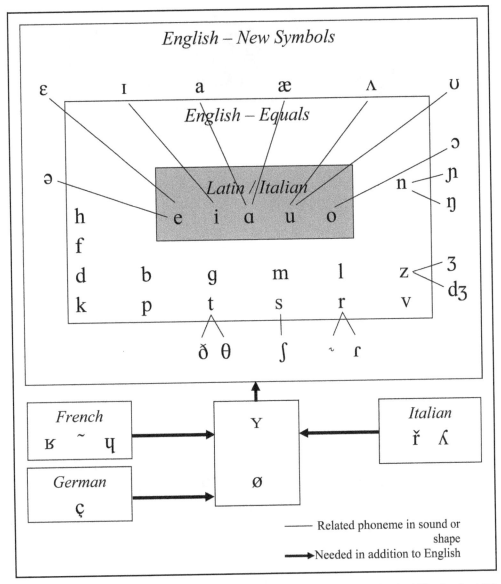

Figure 5–1. Familiar International Phonetic Alphabet table from *The Craft of Singing* (p. 187) by Garyth Nair. Copyright © 2007 Plural Publishing, Inc. All Rights Reserved.

sponding gum ridges. (Those who are interested in learning more about the science of the acoustics should consult Miller, 1986; Nair, 2007; Stevens, 2000; Sundberg, 1987; Titze, 2000.)

In Chapter 2, we saw that the tongue is our most malleable resonator and will go into more detail later in the book. Every vowel phoneme has its own unique tongue shape, but in all of them, the airway remains open. For instance, when you open your mouth and gently flick a finger on your cheek or "cluck" your tongue (do not make a sound with your vocal folds), you will

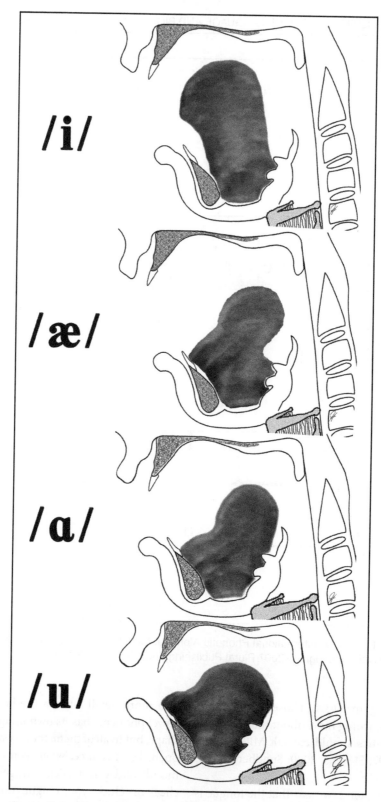

Figure 5–2. Ultrasound-derived sagittal images of sung vowel shapes applying the low mandible maneuver.

hear the air resonating a "pitch" in your oral (mouth) and pharyngeal (throat) cavities. The manipulation of the space with the tongue is important from both an overall resonant (Chapter 3) as well as a phonemic point of view.

Formants

The adjustment of your tongue while doing this exercise changed both the timbre and pitch of the resonance. You may ask, "why is that"? In Chapter 3, we talked about the semioccluded vocal tract (SOVT) or a semienclosed airspace. Remember, we are a three-dimensional structure; thus, our vocal tract is like a tube that has its own frequency. What does that mean? Let us have a look at another example. Did you ever blow across a bottle's top and make a wonderful, resonant sound? This is because the sound travels in and out of the bottle. But here is the puzzle piece we want to tune in right now. Dependent on the geometry of the bottle—various lengths, diameters, volumes, and so on—it will, for instance, give us a high pitch (more water in the bottle or a shorter bottle) or a low pitch (little water in bottle or long bottle). In Figure 5–3, you can see that our vocal tract has a variety of areas such as the oral resonance and pharyngeal resonance chambers.

Now imagine, you are standing on top of the mountain (lips), about to enter a cave (your vocal tract) to explore the various chambers, only now they are morphed and shaped by our articulators (passive and active) and various cavities (oral, pharyngeal, etc.) instead of stalactites (icicle-shaped formation that hangs from the ceiling), stalagmites (opposite of stalactites, project upward), columns, and so on. The diameter at your lips may start to be wide, and you can stand upright, followed by a little narrowing from your teeth where you need to

duck a little (almost like stalactites hanging down). Though when you look between the lips and teeth, there is a little wider crack before the diameter decreases again. Next, continue with a knee-crawl through an even narrower space between the tongue and the small protuberance just behind the upper front teeth (alveola ridge) before you can walk upright and stretch your arms in the higher palate region. Keep in mind that you need to stay very much in the center of your tube, since the sides only lead to tiny cracks with sharp rocks (upper and lower teeth) and a downward slope of the palate.

Do you start to see the picture? Now, we all have our own personal dimensions and shapes of our vocal tract; thus, we have a certain resonant frequency determined by the various parameters (length, diameters, volumes, etc.). This is why two women singing the same pitch and vowel have a different sound. Similar to a person who has an identity document (ID) that proves that person's identity, so has our vocal tract a specific ID, only now we call it resonant frequency instead of date of birth, fingerprints, and so on. However, unlike a fingerprint, we are able to manipulate our parameters of the vocal tract by changing the shape and concomitant diameter, length, and so on, with our active articulators, such as the tongue. This enables us, for instance, to create various vowel sounds (see Figure 5–2), as you heard when you gently flicked on your cheek while changing tongue positions.

Depending on the adjustment, the resonator seems to favor certain frequencies depending on its acoustic parameters. These resonating frequencies in the vocal tract are called *formants*. They are areas in our vocal tract that can acoustically sympathize with the harmonics passing through them, resulting in a boost in amplitude. Other harmonics that do not pass through a sympathetic formant frequency are either

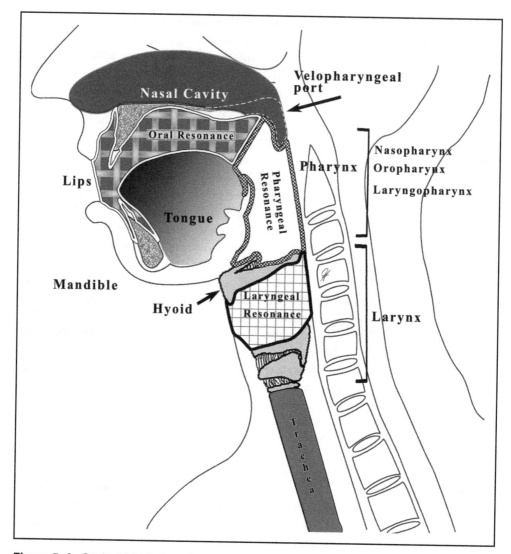

Figure 5–3. Sagittal (side) view of various resonance cavities.

attenuated or even canceled out. Because of the formants, we are able to perceive differences between instruments and individuals and are able to understand different language sounds in both speech and song.

The tongue, however, is not the only part that can change the formants. The articulators—typically the tongue, lips, teeth, palate, and mandible—in various combinations, form all the phonemes that we speak or sing (Figure 5–4). We can divide them into

- *active,* or lower articulators, such as the tongue, lower teeth, lower lip, mandible; and
- *passive,* or upper articulators, such as the upper lip, teeth, upper (alveolar) gum ridge. One could also make the case that the upper lip can be active as well.

Later in the book we delve into the "how" of using those articulators (Chap-

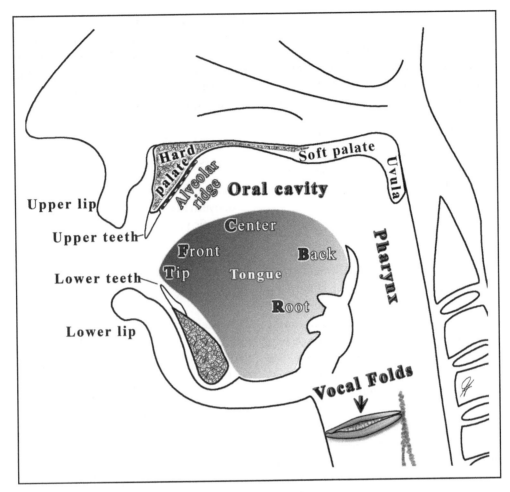

Figure 5–4. Left midsagittal image showing the articulators.

ter 7), the various combinations, and their manipulation, particularly for consonance (Part II).

Source Filter Theory

As discussed in Chapter 3, without our vocal tract resonator, as well as the ability to reshape it, we would only hear the harmonic series of the complex periodic vibration of our vocal folds and one timbre from the voice. The formants affect the acoustic spectrum produced by the vibrating (oscil-lating) vocal folds, which is a phenomenon that can be explained by the **source-filter theory**. *In this theory, the sound source is the time-varying glottal airflow, and the filter is the vocal tract. Whereas the glottis produces a sound of many frequencies, the vocal tract selects (filters) a subset of these frequencies for radiation from the mouth* (Titze, 2000).

Just like any filter, the function enables something to pass through and prevents anything else. In our case, we have an acoustical filtering system that enhances some harmonic frequencies, lets others pass through without change, and hinders others.

In Figure 5–5, you can see

- the source signal produced by the vibrating vocal folds (thin vertical lines simulated from research data);
- the formants (stubby "mountain peaks") shaped by the vocal tract resonator (vocal tract and articulators, which are the movable parts of our anatomical structures, such as the musculature in the walls of the pharynx or the tongue); and
- the radiated signal leaving the mouth (gray peaks).

You can see that those formants (frequency areas of the resonator labeled F_1, F_2, and F_3) only enhance the amplitude of the harmonic frequencies of the source signal that coincide with them. Conversely, in areas where there is no formant, the amplitude peaks of the radiated signal are lower than those found in the source signal.

All of this means that while you sustain on a sung pitch (e.g., A_4 = **source**), the harmonic series stays constant. The moment you change one of the physical resonators (e.g., tongue, lips, etc. = **filter**), the "mountain peaks" (formants) will change and subsequently alter the radiated signal (gray peaks) with it.

The formants are numbered in the order of their frequencies with the label F and a subscript identifying number. In the vocal tract, there are at least five important formants present and working:

- F_1 → basically in the pharynx
- F_2 → mostly in the mouth (oral cavity)
- F_3 "personal timbre" ⎫
- F_4 "the tone and ring" ⎬ Singer's Formant
- F_5 of the voice" ⎭

The first two formants, F_1 and F_2, are essential to the identification of the vowel

one is speaking or singing. Then F_3 and F_4 contain most of the information responsible for our unique vocal timbre. Everything from F_5 and above conveys the "ring" in the voice. The upper frequencies give the voice the fire and brilliance that help project into large or acoustically poor rooms.

The "functionality" of these formants can serve and be looked at in various ways:

- I can reshape my vocal tract (through my active articulators) in order to create a specific phoneme (vowel, consonant) or
- I can reshape my vocal tract through the shape of a particular vowel, such as /i/ (as in k<u>ee</u>n) to change the color and/or dynamic of the sound.

We tend to think of articulatory maneuvers for intelligibility reasons only. However, that is just one slice of the entire voice production cake. By filtering different harmonics, we can change the vowel or its acoustic properties. For instance, more often than not, the intuitive reaction of a singer or actor is to change the source (vocal folds) by pushing harder or the like, to accomplish either more intensity (loudness) and/or brassiness in the sound because the decoupling of source and filter (vocal tract) is not yet established. This is why—besides laryngeal position, lip formation, and jaw position—the tongue is a crucial part in terms of source-filter interaction. Its highly selective and malleable characteristics (Chapter 2) allow us to fine-tune in terms of vowel modification and/or voice quality. Changing the shape of the tongue concomitantly changes the vocal tract's shape and thus the filter (see Chapter 7).

Perception Versus Physiology

Theoretically, the source-filter theory is relatively easy to understand. The difficulty

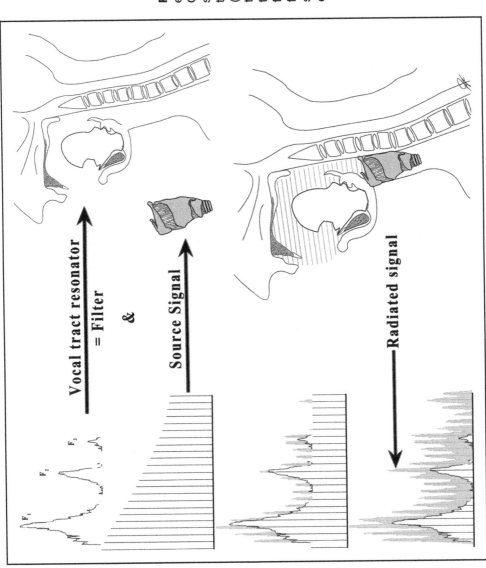

Figure 5–5. A radiated vocal sound and the effect in producing a specific radiated signal. On the left is a gradual overlay of the power spectra, showing the effect of the formants on the harmonic amplitude of the source signal (*bottom*). On the right, we can see the vocal tract resonator shaped to the characteristics of the vowel /i/ (*top*), leaving only certain areas for the frequencies of the source signal (vocal folds) to resonate (*bottom*). Once the radiated spectrum passes through the "filter," the listeners hear the radiated signal (*gray areas*).

starts once students begin to consciously put the theory into practice. One of the biggest obstacles they encounter is differentiating between perception and physiology. This is a sensible subject, though I hope this little discussion will bring some light into the controversy and make it much easier on the singer/actor to establish his or her personal instrument.

First, what is it that we want to accomplish?

The goal is to gradually decouple the control of various **filter changes** (in other words, the articulators, particularly the tongue) from the actual **sound production** (voice box) *and* the **tactile feedback** (that is, the vibrational feedback in the face, often referred to as "mask").

One hears singers, actors, teachers, coaches, directors, and conductors repeatedly guiding peers and clients to "sing into the mask" or "place their voice in the mask." Their help is well-intended but, unfortunately, more often than not, based on false facts, myths, and mainly solely on their personal perception (without knowledge of the physiology). While the sensation of various vibrations in the face is part of our feedback in singing/speaking, it has nothing to do with the anatomy and physiology of singing/speaking itself.

As described in Chapter 2, the vocal tract and its anatomical apparatus is an intricately connected and finely tuned instrument. Thus, for example, changing the tongue body position and shape without raising, stiffening, or tensing up the voice box (larynx) is very hard at first. However, as in any skill, learning—no matter if it is singing, speaking, sports, juggling, and so on—requires the acquisition of motor patterns.

Because singing or speaking happens out of sight—inside of our body, and unconscious/involuntary—before taking any training, we need biofeedback, such as ultrasound (see later), as an indispensable technique to learn how to control internal functions. Also, our kinesthetic and tactile feedback is much more reliable than our internal auditory feedback because singing/speaking is a lie. What does that bold statement mean? Do you remember the first time you heard your voice recorded on a device, like an answering machine? I assume the reaction was something like, "No, do I really sound like that!?" The reasons are because (a) we hear our voice via the bones of the skull, which is why it sounds louder to us; and (b) the sound quality we perceive internally is considerably altered (the bones reduce the high-frequency components of the sound, and the radiated sound from the mouth reaches our ear as reflected sound). This is also why you should not listen to yourselves, because you may think you are aiming for a certain sound, when in fact you are going for a lie.

Finally, let us not forget the incumbent acoustic challenges of most spaces in which we have to perform, where the perception/our own biofeedback of our singing/speaking is the only constant we can count on. So, we need to be careful in discerning what we perceive and how we re-create the feedback.

So, what kind of feedback are we talking about? We have two classes of feedback: kinesthetic and tactile. The gross, simplified definitions are as follows:

Kinesthetic feedback
Represents that which you feel from sensors in your muscles, joints, tendons. For instance, information like the distance and angle of your jaw opening, the stretch and position of your tongue

in, for example the vowel /i/, within your mouth is given to your brain.

Tactile feedback

is represented by sensations you feel on your surface. For instance, the vibration within your face, under the skin (often referred to as "mask")

Remember how the filter (our resonators/articulators) radiates certain frequencies and quasi-dampens others? Let us look at this from a different perspective. In Figure 5–6, you can see the picture of one of the most wonderful looking *and* sounding concert halls on the east coast of the United States: The Concert Hall at Drew University, Madison, New Jersey (to read more about the acoustics and the story of the hall, please visit: http://www.drew.edu/news/2013/03/12/looks-beautiful-sounds-beautiful [retrieved October 2018]). When building a concert hall, one has to consider the size and shape of the room as well as various reflecting surfaces (materials and angles) on which the sound bounces off. One acoustic feature in this hall is the **acoustical reflector** on the ceiling, known as "the jewel." The piano (source) generates sound waves (indicated by the arrows) that are reflected by the jewel and, depending on where and off what angle they bounce, are redirected into the house, stage, balcony, and so forth, where they continue to reflect.

Let us keep focusing on the jewel, although for our purposes we imagine it upside down. Now, instead of reflecting downward, it will reflect upward, as you might have guessed, just like our tongue. The difference between the jewel and the tongue is that the former is preset and inflexible, and the latter, variable and flexible. When continuing to follow Figure 5–6 clockwise, you can see various tongue posi-

tions (/i/ = gray; /ɑ/ = black/green; /u/ = violet). Depending on the position and shape of the tongue, the concomitant change of the reflection of the sound waves generated by the vocal folds (source) is the key. Have a look at how the gray arrows for /i/ have very little room between tongue tip/surface and front of the hard palate (remember the "two rooms" depicted in Figure 5–3), while the black/green arrows from /ɑ/ are free to travel around in the very spot because of the different tongue shape. Thus, the reflection of the same sound wave will change as the tongue shape itself changes.

Can you see where this is headed? Let us add one more puzzle piece before we conclude with the end result. I am sure you have seen or even owned a plasma ball (Figure 5–6, bottom middle). The electrode at the center of a plasma ball emits an electric current that displays as colorful tendrils of light. The color depends on the gasses used inside the plasma ball. If you ever touched a plasma ball when it is on, you know that placing your finger on the glass draws a colorful strand of light to your finger. It is like creating your own personal bolt of lightning from the electrode to your finger. This is similar to tactile feedback, the feeling you have in the tip of your finger once connected to a lightning stream.

Last, let us put all the pieces together: imagine that the inside of the plasma ball is your vocal tract (mouth, teeth, tongue, larynx, etc.) set for every phoneme, like the vowel /i/. And then consider that the outside of the ball is your skin and the bones of your face, giving you tactile feedback in the form of vibrations. You will learn to use your kinesthetic feedback to sense how to stretch or move your tongue in order to set up the vowel. Now, the anatomical and physiological setup of the phoneme determines how the sound will bounce off and reflect

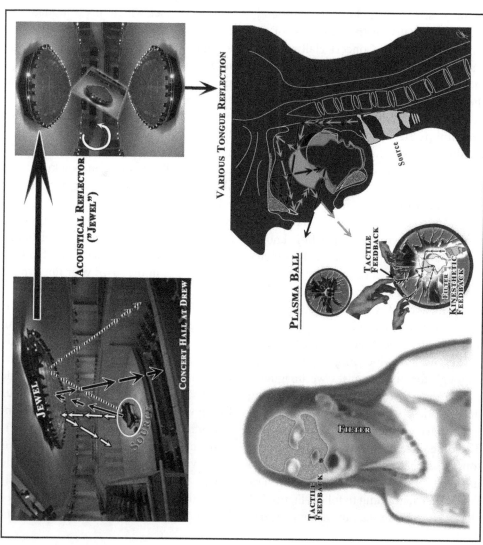

Figure 5–6. *Upper left corner:* Large acoustical reflector ("jewel") directs sound back to the house and stage. *Upper right corner:* Imagine the jewel turned upside down, now reflecting upward, like the tongue in the lower right corner. In the lower middle, a plasma ball emits high frequencies from the center (like the sound wave reflection from the tongue) that reflect on the surface (like the vibration on the skin) when touched. The vibration on the skin (either pinpointed or areas) is the tactile feedback we feel. Depending on the position and setup of the tongue, this tactile feedback (often referred to as "mask") changes because the reflections are redirected. Thus, the anatomical use of the filter (tongue, larynx, etc.) is independent from the sensation one feels in the face/skull.

within the space. As a result, the sound will bounce off and reflect differently on each vowel/phoneme, which in turn—and here is the "biggie"—will create different sensations on the skin surface and bones of your face.

Looking at the singer in Figure 5–6, you see the word "Filter," referring to the tongue positions inside, and a gray/green colored area in the face, where certain vibrations may be sensed. These may sometimes be wider spread and/or pinpointed. Coming back to the "singing into the mask" statement, if one instructs a singer to "place" the voice in a certain spot on the face, most of the time it ends up with the singer trying to push the sound into that particular direction. Consequently, the larynx, the tongue, and so forth, tense up and push forward. However, if one works with the singer to first generate sound without strain and, second, find the ideal tongue position for the vowel /i/, they learn through kinesthetic feedback to use the voice box (larynx) and tongue independently. Once that is established (meaning the filter is set), only then should the singer begin to connect that setup to the vibration in the face (tactile feedback), in other words, feeling the result of sound reflections in the face and not placing the voice in the mask. This process has to be established *individually* because even though anatomically we are similar, the size, proportions, and so forth, are different and therefore create different reflections, hence different vibration "in the mask." This is why I like to work on the manipulation of the articulators one by one or choose that which requires most attention first—it is highly probable that it is the tongue; another "perception versus physiology" in itself, due to its hydrostatic nature (Chapters 2 and 6). Once the student reaches or gets close to the "ideal." I always ask, "How does it feel?" to build up both kinesthetic and tactile feedback. Ultimately, fine singers and actors will

eventually rely on a combination of how the vocal production feels, coupled with internal and external acoustic clues.

Closed Vocal Tract

Consonants, in general, involve some degree of obstruction in the form of closure or near-closure of the vocal tract. Saying each of the consonants /k/, /p/, and /g/ involves a momentary complete blockage of the airway with either the tongue or the lips. Because of that momentary closure, the airway is considered closed, even if just for a split second.

Now, say these consonants from another phonemic class, /s/, /ʃ/, and /f/. Notice that even though there is no complete blockage of airflow, your articulators (teeth and/or lips) allow only a miniscule gap through which air can flow. This tiny aperture causes the airflow to become turbulent and create noise. This "almost-stoppage" is also considered a closed vocal tract because the action can be sustained (try it out: it is easy to sustain a /ʃ/ for 5 sec or more).

In consonants, the articulators correspond with a **place of articulation (PoA)**, from the front of the vocal tract to the back (Figure 5–7). The more mobile parts of the vocal tract, such as lips and tongue, are **active PoAs** contrary to the **passive PoAs** that constitute parts anywhere from the upper teeth, gums, or roof of the mouth to the back of the throat.

To elaborate on Figure 5–7:

Labials: Sounds are produced by one or both lips.

Dentals: Tongue contacts the teeth.

Alveolar: Tongue contacts the area behind the upper teeth.

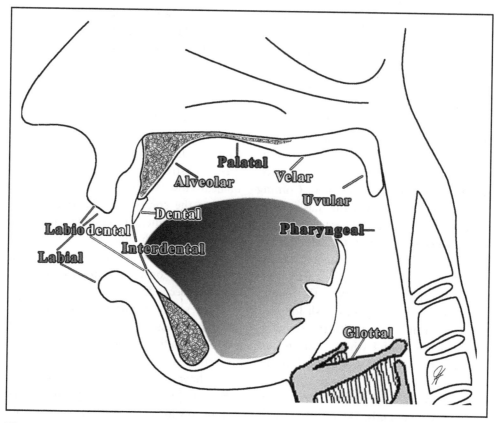

Figure 5–7. The relationships between the articulators and their corresponding places of articulation.

Palatal: Tongue contacts part of the hard palate, or roof of the mouth. Because the palate is relatively large, it can be divided into **alveopalatals**, **prepalatals, palatals,** and **postpalatals**.

Velar: Tongue contacts the soft palate (velum).

Glottal: Does not have an actual PoA but uses partial adduction of the vocal folds for some friction or turbulence.

We discuss a far more complete definition of consonants later in this book. However, to complete the introduction into the building blocks of language, we ought to mention one more descriptive subdivision:

voicing or **phonation**. We are talking about various voiced sounds that require phonation: a process initiated by airflow, in which the vocal folds are vibrating (oscillation)— opening (abduction) and closing (adduction) the space between the vocal folds (glottis), and producing vocal sound and speech. As long as this pressurized air continues to flow through the narrowed glottis, phonation will be sustained. These vibratory cycles are extremely fast, for example, reaching 440 times a second when singing a middle A.

Unless we are whispering, all the vowels are voiced. The consonants, on the other hand, can be broadly categorized into two classes:

▨ can be sustained and sung on pitch and

▨ are pure noise and do not have a pitch component.

The former we classify as **"consovowels"** (consonant plus vowel), adapting the definition from Garyth Nair (2007). He expanded the term, originally coined by Henderson and Palmer (1940, p. 356), and only included the phonemes /m, n, ŋ, l, and r/, to include *all* consonants that can be executed on pitch (Chapter 7).

Last, but not least, along the voicing and point of articulation, we have the **manner of articulation (MoA)**. This classification of consonants now refers to *how* the sound is produced. Sometimes, the positioned articulator (PoA) will stop the airflow completely, or the blockage will only be partial. In other words, the MoA relates to the acoustic properties of the consonants. The most common MoAs for consonants are **obstruents** (stops, fricatives, affricates, stridents, sibilants) and **sonorants** (approximants, nasals, laterals, liquids, glides). But again, more on that is presented later (Chapter 7).

Ultrasound as Biofeedback

Ultrasound has been proven as a noninvasive instrument, primarily used by healthcare professionals to view the heart, blood vessels, kidneys, liver, and other organs. Maureen Stone of the University of Maryland originally developed the technique of the acquisition of midsagittal (midline slice) tongue profiles. Her research primarily focused on finding strategies that can be adapted after a tongue cancer surgery (glossectomy) where part of the tongue is removed.

For the pilot study of the low mandible maneuver (LMM) research, we modified and refined Stone's technique. Ultrasound is an extremely valuable tool in exploring tongue surface activity during singing and speech. Voice pedagogy already uses eye-body biofeedback in the form of virtual real-time spectrography (Miller, 2008; Nair, 1999, 2007), and ultrasound has been successfully used as biofeedback in both clinical settings (Bernhardt, Gick, Bacsfalvi, & Adler-Bock, 2005, Gick, Wilson, and Derrick, 2013) and the language classroom (Honikman, 1964). It was thus a short leap for me—something that might fall under the category of a "no-brainer"—to pioneer the use of ultrasound as biofeedback in the voice studio, workshops, and master classes with impressive success. Additionally, a first-prize-winning poster presentation (Nair & Nair, 2013) and a more recent case study (Nair, Schellenberg, & Gick, 2015) support the view that ultrasound is a tool that has much promise in the voice studio.

I developed techniques and found indications, which are now the basis of this book, that help with mastering a conscious and precise maneuvering/manipulation of the tongue. For example, to overcome the challenges of consonants and vowels, we need to study the relationship of what the singer/actor does physically (tongue physiology) and the acoustic end result the audience hears. The use of ultrasound to analyze tongue motions (Nair et al., 2016; Stone et al., 2005) allows for real-time videos of singers in individual phoneme production and phoneme-to-phoneme transitions during the LMM.

So how do we read those images and videos? In Figure 5–8, you can see an ultrasound image embedded in a sagittal profile (from the right side) with the transducer positioned under the jaw (mandible), and a water reservoir (standoff; see Chapter 6, Figure 6–10) in between. Crystals in the transducer emanate ultrahigh-frequency

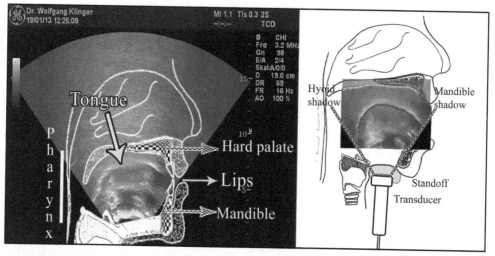

Figure 5–8. Sagittal (from the side) profile embedded in ultrasound image (*left*) and ultrasound image embedded in a sagittal (from the side) profile (right). The back of the tongue (posterior) appears on the left. (Image from Nair & Nair, 2013; Nair et al., 2016.)

sound waves and produce an image by using their reflective properties, showing the tongue surface in real time. The two bones, hyoid on the left and mandible on the right, cast an acoustic shadow on both sides, generating a loss of the extreme tip of the tongue (extreme anterior apex). For the sake of completion, I have to mention that this reflection of the tongue surface represents only a midline slice of the tongue. We are only looking at a two-dimensional structure, where in fact the tongue is obviously a three-dimensional organ. We will go deeper into this subject in Chapter 6. However, for simplicity sake, we continue to talk about the side (sagittal) profile.

At first, this might appear more complicated than it actually is, but do not worry. I have found that after a few minutes of introduction (sometimes less than a minute), students very quickly familiarize themselves with the tongue contour and start to learn to control its movement. Let us have a look at Figure 5–9, which shows two views of the same side (sagittal) image

of the tongue (vowel /i/, from speech). The plain image is on the left, and in the right image, the surface of the tongue is outlined in white/blue. Once students start to follow the contours of the tongue in real time on the screen as they sing/speak, they are surprised to see how fast, complex, and fun it is to monitor the acrobatic nature of the tongue (so much so, that it is sometimes difficult to get them to focus on the task at hand).

As we just mentioned in our little excursion regarding biofeedback: skill learning—whether singing, speaking, sports, or juggling—requires the acquisition of motor patterns. We need biofeedback, such as ultrasound, as an indispensable technique to learn how to control internal functions. This is exactly why it is my sincere belief that ultrasound will become imperative in the future of voice pedagogy. However, it would be financially unreasonable to expect voice pedagogues/coaches to buy their own portable ultrasound machine. The solution to this problem lies in the development of

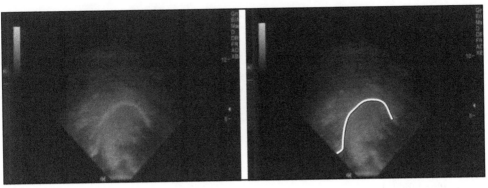

Figure 5–9. Side (sagittal) view of the tongue with ultrasound (vowel /i/). The tip (apex) is on the right and the back of the tongue on the left. The outline is shown in white/blue in the image on the right.

USB ultrasound transducers that can be used directly with any Windows/Mac computer (laptop, tablet, or desktop). As I write, I am working on the development of (a) a USB ultrasound transducer that meets the necessary specifications of a minimum of 30fps and can be used directly with any Windows/Mac device and (b) a possible combination of the ultrasound with real-time spectrum analyses within one software program, avoiding the need for multiple devices and applications.

But, as you will soon see for yourself, even with only the imagery derived from ultrasound, combined with step-by-step instructions, I already experience a rapid acceleration in my students' understanding of the complex vocal strategies such as LMM, tongue shapes, and consonant resonance (Chapter 7). It is my hope that this book will make this knowledge accessible to all, singers and actors alike (an actor faces similar challenges and needs to, for example, project Shakespeare as well as a classical singer does Rossini), and possibly help speech-language pathologists to adapt their approach when working with that clientele—and maybe other populations, too.

References

Bernhardt, B. M., Gick, B., Bacsfalvi, P., & Adler-Bock, M. (2005). Ultrasound in speech therapy with adolescents and adults. *Clinical Linguistics and Phonetics, 19,* 605–617.

Gick, B., Wilson, I., & Derrick, D. (2013). *Articulatory phonetics.* Malden, MA: Wiley-Blackwell.

Henderson, C., & Palmer, C. (1940). *How to sing for money.* New York, NY: Harcourt, Brace.

Honikman, B. (1964). Articulatory settings. In D. Abercrombie, D. B. Fry, P. A. D. MacCarthy, N. C. Scott, & J. L. M. Trim (Eds.), *In honor of Daniel Jones* (pp. 73–84). London, UK: Longmans.

Miller, R. (1986). *The structure of singing.* New York, NY: Schirmer.

Nair, G. (1999). *Voice, tradition and technology.* San Diego, CA: Singular Publishing.

Nair, A., & Nair, G. (2013). *Ultrasound: Tracking tongue profiles and resonance creation in the singing voice.* Poster presented at the Annual Symposium: Care of the Professional Voice, The Voice Foundation, Philadelphia, PA. Awarded Best Poster 2013.

Nair, A., Nair, G., & Reishofer, G. (2016). The low mandible maneuver and its resonential implications for elite singers. *Journal of Voice, 30,* 128.e13–128.e32.

Nair, A., Schellenberg, M., & Gick, B. (2015). A case study on the efficacy of ultrasound biofeedback in voice pedagogy. In The Scottish Consortium for ICPhS 2015 (Ed.), *Proceedings of the 18th International Congress of Phonetic Sciences (ICPhS)*, University of Glasgow, Scotland, UK. London, UK: International Phonetic Association. https://www.internationalphoneticassociation.org/icphs-proceedings/ICPhS2015/proceedings.html

Nair, G. (2007). *The craft of singing.* San Diego, CA: Plural Publishing.

Stevens, K. N. (2000). *Acoustic phonetics.* Cambridge, MA: MIT Press.

Stone, M. (2005). A guide to analyzing tongue motion from ultrasound images. *Clinical Linguistics Phonetics, 19,* 455–502.

Sundberg, J. (1987). *The science of the singing voice.* Dekalb, IL: Northern Illinois University Press.

Titze, I. (2000). *Principles of voice production* (2nd ed.). Iowa City, IA: National Center for Voice and Speech.

6 Vowels and Vowels That You Thought Were Consonants

A Chapter on Vowels in a Book About Consonants?

Having covered phonetics and resonance, we are almost ready to tackle the central subject of this book: consonant resonance. However, if we are going to have any hope of granting our consonants "resonantial parity" with our vowels, we have to make sure we understand how great singing vowels or "say it as a singer" (SAS) vowels with good resonance work. Then, and only then, we can focus on the consonants in order to create the singing line we desire. However, for more detailed instructions on how to learn the proper vowels, I would like to refer you to Garyth Nair's *The Craft of Singing* (2007).

Most vocal pedagogy literature has generally looked to the speech field for its phonetic information. However, singing is not speech; therefore, book after book misses some needed information based on what singers actually do (not all, but way too many do).

In most vocal pedagogy literature, the vowels are presented as listed in Table 6–1.

Front, Back, and Central Vowels

Notice that the vowels listed in Table 6–1 are divided into three basic categories: front, central, and back. These designations are

Table 6–1. Table of Standard Vowels

Front		Central	Back	
i	see		u	boot
ɪ	sit		ʊ	book
ʏ	Gr. umlaut ü		o	moan
e	say			
ɛ	set	ə Schwa	ɔ	open It. o
ø	Gr. umlaut ö		ʌ	up
æ	sat		ʊ	foot
a	father		ɑ	law

based on *where* the tongue is when it divides the oral cavity in two. To employ our "two-rooms-connected-by-a-hallway" metaphor, when the tongue is in the front (anterior), it is considered a **front vowel**—the smaller resonance space is in the front, and the larger is in the back. The **back vowels** are the reverse—the tongue is moved back on the frontal (coronal) plane so that the larger resonance space is in the front.

Figure 6–1 shows the tongue shapes from a side view (sagittal view) of the back vowel /ɑ/ and the front vowel /i/. Note the differences of space between the front of the tongue and the hard palate/teeth (alveolar ridge).

Before we continue to look into the three-dimensional (3D) perspective of the tongue, let us remind ourselves that the tongue is a muscular hydrostat whose most important biomechanical feature is that it is volume preserving. As discussed in Chapters 2 and 5, both the vowel classifications as well as common directional instructions (e.g., "move the tongue forward or back") are kinesthetically not beneficial for the singer/actor because being a muscular hydrostat means that every movement of the tongue is accompanied by deformation. Thus, the two-dimensional (2D) shapes you are seeing are composed of simultaneously occur-

ring retractions and extensions rather than the displacement of the entire tongue.

For a better understanding on how to read the following 3D images and recognize the sometimes minimal but very subtle changes of tongue shapes, we look at the following graph adapted after the segmentation by Stone and Lundberg (1996).

Until now, we always referred to the shape of the tongue, and the vocal tract for that matter, as a 2D structure. Three-dimensional reconstructions of the tongue's surface are difficult to acquire through current technology, such as magnetic resonance imaging (MRI), computed tomography (CT), and ultrasound (US) (Stone & Lundberg, 1996). Although we continue to refer to 2D images, there are certain indications in 2D images that will help us determine whether some 3D characteristics are present or not.

For a thorough understanding of the range and complexity of tongue shapes, the classification of vowel categories and consonants, as well as a more complete interpretation of 2D images, we need to look at 3D tongue surface shapes. Let us start with Stone and Lundberg's (1996) description of the segments of the tongue (Figure 6–2).

This is easily seen in Figure 6–3, which shows a front and back vowel with the

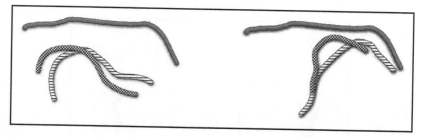

Figure 6–1. Two sagittal tongue shapes for the vowels /ɑ/ (*left*) and /i/ (*right*) that were derived from ultrasound data. The checkered/red lines show the tongue shape by a professional singer (with a dropped mandible platform), and the striped/green lines are the same person's speech profiles. The gray/yellow line represents the hard palate.

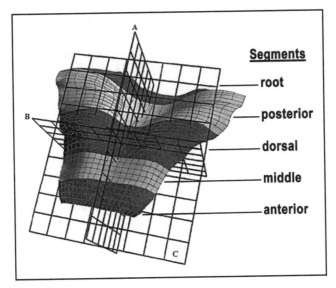

Figure 6–2. The five lengthways segments of the tongue described by Stone (1990) and Stone and Lundberg (1996). Image courtesy of the Acoustical Society of America.

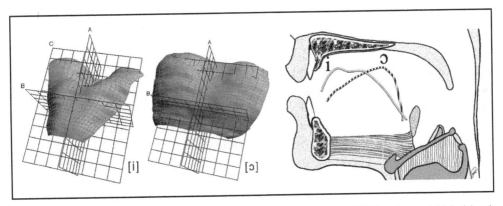

Figure 6–3. Comparison of typical front and back vowel shapes. (left) front vowel /i/; (m) back vowel open "o" (/ɔ/), (right) sagittal views of the two shapes (*gray/red* = /i/ and *striped/green* = /ɔ/). Three-dimensional tongue shapes from Stone and Lundberg (1996). Images courtesy of the Acoustical Society of America.

tongue in three dimensions as well as in a sagittal view (from the side).

Stone and Lundberg (1996) found that the tongue uses a limited repertoire of surface shapes for most English phonemes and classified it using four different categories: (a) front raising, (b) complete groove, (c) back raising, and (d) two-point displacement. In addition, **electropalatography** (EPG)[1] revealed three tongue-palate contact

---

[1]A custom-made artificial plate monitors contact between tongue and hard palate.

patterns: (a) bilateral (two-sided) contact, (b) crosswise contact, and (c) a combination of the two. Both vowels and consonants seemed to use similar tongue shapes but differ in vocal tract location. However, consonants interact with the hard palate and therefore create an additional sound source by manipulating the vocal tract shape. We discuss the importance and impact of the different surface shapes in more detail later.

Before looking at more tongue shapes, it is important to keep in mind that we are primarily looking at 2D images. This might suffice for a basic description of vowels in speech; however, with the increase of oropharyngeal space through the low mandible maneuver (LMM), even vowels become a more complex 3D model of intrinsic, extrinsic tongue and jaw muscles—as we discuss in more detail later in this chapter. We already know that because of the hydrostatic nature of the tongue (Chapter 2), the volume is constant. So, when we talk about tongue shapes, we need to look at both 2D (up-down, front-back) and 3D (elongation, various distinct regions of contraction or expansion) shapes. Since most of the imagery used in this book is derived from ultrasound, we are confined to looking at 2D images.

Front Vowels

In a **front vowel**, the apex of the tongue is forward in the oral cavity. In our two-room/hallway metaphor, this configuration creates a small "room" in the front of the oral cavity and a large "room" in the back. Figure 6–4 shows the common front vowels in a 3D representation of speech configurations (the singing configurations will be different because of the dropped mandible platform).

Notice how the entire tongue gradually relaxes in these images from the left to the right as the midline groove deepens (plane A).

Also, beginning with the /i/ vowel at the left, the apex (the highest point of the vertical curve) of the tongue runs totally across the tongue, but as one moves toward the right and the midline groove deepens, you will see that the tongue edges retain a convexity near plane B.

Let us have a look at the same series of vowels seen in the 3D speech shapes (see Figure 6–4) that can be seen in a series of ultrasound-derived surface shapes (in Figure 6–5). They clearly show the apex of the tongue moving as it divides the resonance space.

This book is all about the effect of the drop of the mandible platform on the resonance of the classical singer. It is now time to have a more detailed look at the effect of the LMM on the tongue of the singer. The same speech shapes given in Figure 6–5 are shown again in Figure 6–6, but now, the singing tongue shape needed with the mandible down is superimposed on the speech shape (gray/red lines). (Incidentally, these shapes were derived from ultrasounds of the same subject.)

Notice how the singer's tongue surface in those gray/red tracings reshapes so that more resonance space is created either by shifting the tongue tip (apex) and/or by creating more space, sometimes both anteriorly and posteriorly. Additionally, you can see how often the posterior space is increased. This is of critical importance because it couples with the increased length and breadth of the pharynx partially enabled by the dropped mandible.

It should be noted that it is possible that the speech profiles shown here and in the following chapters are those of a trained, professional singer and are therefore better than those of the average voice user.

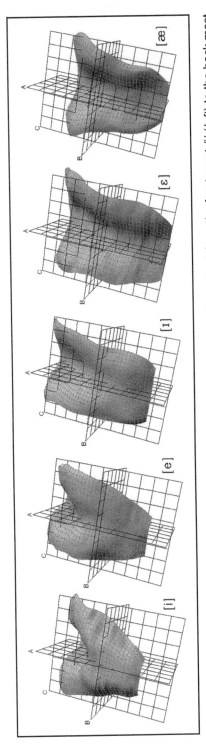

Figure 6–4. Three-dimensional images of the front vowel series (in speech configuration) from the front-most /i/ (*left*) to the back-most /æ/ (*right*). Three-dimensional tongue shapes from Stone and Lundberg (1996). Images courtesy of the Acoustical Society of America.

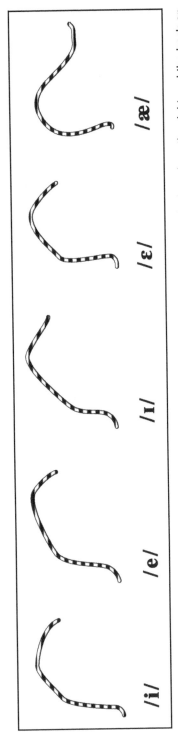

Figure 6–5. The front vowels' sagittal speech forms (derived from ultrasound images) with the tip (apex) on the right and the back on the left.

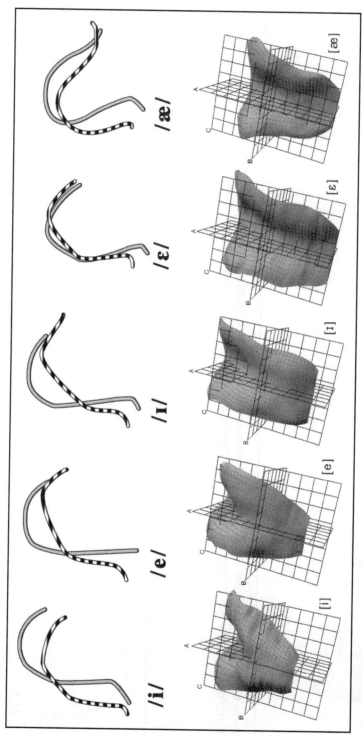

Figure 6–6. The speech vowel tongue shapes shown in Figure 6–5 are now overlain with the tongue shape necessitated by the low mandible (*gray/red*). The three-dimensional shapes from Figure 6–4 are shown again so the reader can compare the shapes.

At a certain point in the habituation of increased resonance, the singing technique seems also to impact on speech (Lee et al., 2008). Most professional singers have had the experience of someone they do not know approaching them at a party, saying "Where did you study voice?" One resonance creator knows the telltale sounds of another.

The tongue surface has already shown us the various changes within the front vowels. To help visualize it even better, let us have a look at the same spoken and sung tongue shapes within the oropharyngeal cavity for a more detailed context, particularly regarding the resonance chambers (Figure 6–7).

The vowel /æ/ is a special case because some texts consider it a central vowel as it sits so low and relatively flat in the oral cavity. Other vowels, such as /ɑ/, also sit low and seem to be almost similar in their 2D shape. So how is it that there is such a difference in not only vowel identification but also timbre? To find the answer to this question, we need to remind ourselves of the hydrostatic nature of the tongue and change the perspective from a sagittal (from the side) to a coronal (from the front) view (see The Groove section later).

Central Vowels

In a central vowel, the apex of the tongue is midway in the oral cavity. This creates relatively equal spaces on either side of the apex of the tongue.

While most pedagogues and scientists easily welcome the schwa (/ə/) as a vowel, they relegate the two relatives of the schwa, the schwar /ɚ/ and the stressed schwar /ɝ/ to the consonant lists because the printed letter "r" is present. However, we take the position, both from the acoustical and physiological viewpoints, that /ɚ/ and /ɝ/ are actually produced as vowels and should be considered as such along with the schwa (Figure 6–8).

Note the similarity in profile of these three phonemes (two "bumps" with a valley in between). The physical differences between the three are mostly the attitude and placement of the characteristic profile.

However, despite the fact that a dropped-too-far mandible will convert the schwa into a pure vowel, do we singers/actors use any drop to get the schwa more resonant? Informal exploration would suggest that we drop the mandible but reduce the angle of the platform (Figure 6–9). This is certainly a good question and may become a separate research paper on its own.

Though based on the analyses of the vast amount of data collected in the LMM study (Nair et al., 2016), the present conjecture is that there is limited mandible drop in the central /ə/. How do we know that? In order to permit and measure jaw movement, we used a standoff (water-filled, acoustically transparent reservoir) between the transducer head and the bottom of the jaw (Figure 6–10 and Chapter 5, Figure 5–8). As a result, the size and shape of the fluid reservoir at the bottom of the wedge seen in the ultrasound (see Figure 6–10) indicate both how much the mandible has dropped and the angle. In this example, the drop for the sung /ə/ measures about 0.75 mm (by way of comparison, front and back vowels can show a drop between 1 and 2.5 cm). Also, notice how the left side (posterior, back of the tongue) of the concave curve is lower than the right (anterior, front side of the tongue).

In addition, a picture sequence taken from a video of a separate side-view camera that recorded throughout the protocol confirms those findings (Figure 6–11).

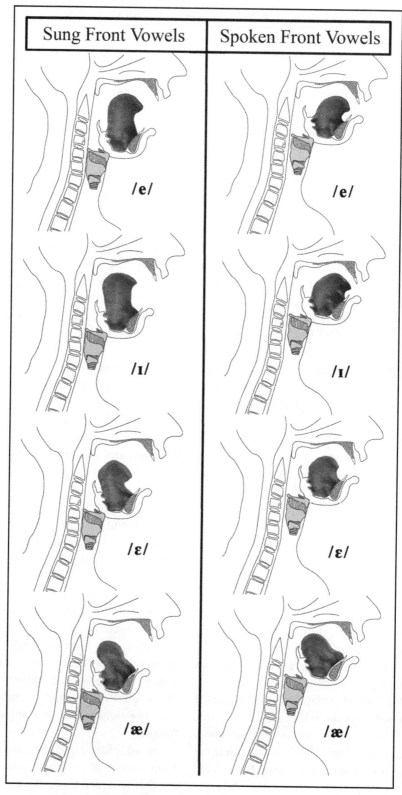

Figure 6–7. Contrasting juxtaposition of sung (using the first strategy of the low mandible maneuver) and spoken front vowels.

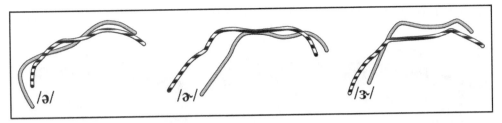

Figure 6–8. The central vowels; speech is shown in striped/blue, and gray/red depicts singing.

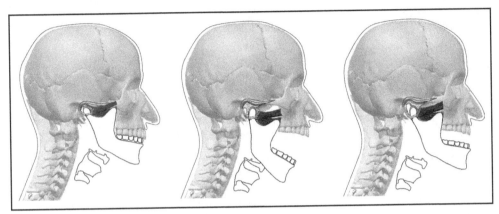

Figure 6–9. Nair theory of mandible drop during schwa production. Mandible up (*left*), full singer mandible drop (*center*), and condyle drop at temporomandibular joint but mandible up for schwa production (*right*).

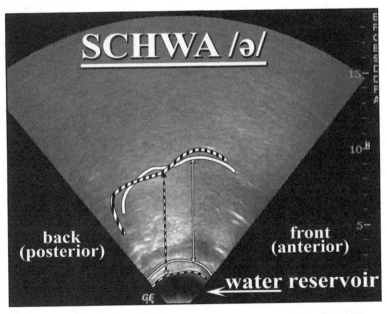

Figure 6–10. Ultrasound of a sung /ə/ (*striped/red*) overlaid with a spoken /ə/ (*white/blue*). Notice the different size and shape of the water reservoir for each /ə/ at the bottom of the wedge. It indicates both the mandible drop for the sung /ə/ as well as the angle tilting posteriorly.

81

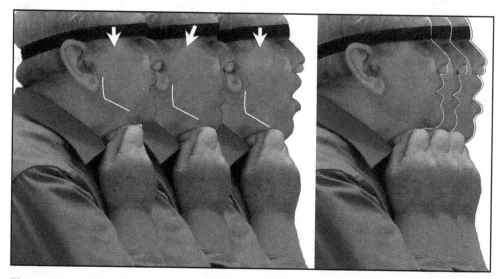

Figure 6–11. Sequence (*left to right*) of the mandible drop and mouth opening during schwa production (spoken and sung) and full low mandible maneuver (LMM) (sung /ɔ/). *Left:* Notice the gradual augmentation of the bulge from the condyle by the subtle shadow change above the cheek (*arrow*) as well as the change of the angle/position of the ramus (*white/yellow* lines). *Right:* compared to the spoken /ə/ (*left*), there is only a slight increase in mouth opening for the sung /ə/ (*middle*) as opposed to the maximum opening on the sung /ɔ/ with full LMM (*right*).

The shadow above the cheek gradually disappears because of the increase of the bulge from the condyle moving forward. However, compared to a full LMM, there is only a minimal movement for the sung /ə/ (indicated by the arrow) though a change in the angle of the ramus (white/yellow lines). Similar observations can be made when looking at the actual mouth opening on the right side of the same sequence: only a slight increase for the sung /ə/ compared to the spoken /ə/ was seen.

Nevertheless, we seem to use a full drop for /ɚ/ and /ɝ/. So, let us explore the principle with a closer look at the /ə/.

The Schwa—Reason for Its Variability

The first of the missing links in our singer's vowel chart is the one that is asterisked and italicized in the Central classification—the schwa.

The origin of the word *schwa* is from the Hebrew word *shva* (שְׁוָא International Phonetic Alphabet (IPA): [ʃva], classical pronunciation: shewa' [ʃəˈwa]), designating the Hebrew niqqud vowel sign shva (two vertical dots written beneath a letter): in Modern Hebrew, it indicates either the phoneme /e/ or the complete absence of a vowel. This refers to the neutral vowel used for unstressed syllables in English, German, and French:

- English—last syllable in "relat<u>ed</u>"
- German—second syllable of "sehe"
- French—"le"

In fact, in English, the schwa is our most-used vowel, yet most singers or native speakers of English for that matter are not even aware of its existence. Yet, we all *speak* thousands of them every single day. The reason for this is that as the sound for an unaccented (not stressed) syllable, they are executed very quickly. How often does one hear a speaker dwell on a weak syllable for some communicative expression?

The word *entertainment* is a good example. The proper IPA transliteration would be as follows:

$$/ɛntɝˈteɪnmənt/$$

Focus on that last unaccented syllable, *-ment*. The upside-down, backward "e" is the IPA symbol for the schwa.

Lack of Awareness

Unfortunately, there are still singers as well as teachers, coaches, and conductors who are not aware of the schwa (physiologically and/or phonetically), and singers end up with acutely nonidiomatic diction in all three languages. Some examples will suffice here—possible mispronunciations of these three exemplar words are shown in Table 6–2.

Tongue Relaxation

Part of the problem can also be inadvertent tongue relaxation. Proper schwa production requires a certain amount of concavity in the tongue that looks like a "groove." (As we see later in this book, this is an essen-tial part of other phonemes, not only the schwa.) This means that muscles (especially the genioglossus) must shape portions of the tongue downward from the neutral position. Any relaxation of the muscles producing the shape will allow the concave portions of the tongue to rise, an act that quickly destroys the unique timbre of the schwa. We continue the "groove" later on in the back vowels and discuss more on how to execute this delicate maneuver with the tongue in Part II.

The most common singing substitute one hears for the schwa is /ʌ/. In Figure 6–12, we can see why—the schwa is a lower profile, so it takes more muscular action to produce and maintain the shape. When the brain allows the tongue to relax, even just slightly, the concavity necessary for the schwa is lost, and the vowel converts into the back vowel, /ʌ/.

Additionally, from an empirical perspective in my voice studio, I frequently encounter singers who have a hard time maintaining that somewhat constrained, almost neutral position of the tongue, since it does not conclude in an extensive directional movement. Without that movement, it feels as if nothing happens at all, almost "neutral," which leaves the singer/actor in a somewhat lost position of seemingly no control. All of this triggers a more pronounced motion to one of the aforementioned vowels.

Table 6–2. Examples of Mispronunciations of the Schwa		
	Improper Unaccented Syllable	*Proper Unaccented Syllable With the Schwa*
English	/rəleɪtɛd/ or /rəleɪtʌd/	rəleɪtəd
German	/zeɛ/ or /zeʌ/	/zeə/
French	/le/, /lʌ/, or /lɛ/	/lə/

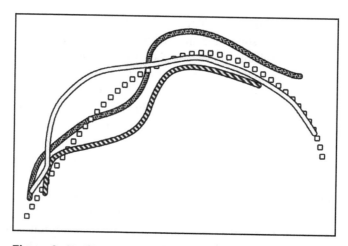

Figure 6–12. The schwa profile /ə/ (*striped/red*) and the commonly substituted pure vowels /ʌ/ (*white/green*) and /ɛ/ (*fishbone/orange*). The at-rest position of the tongue is shown as the dotted line in white/purple.

Too Much Mouth Opening/ Mandible Platform Drop

A third reason that the schwa too easily becomes /ʌ/ is the insidious reason introduced at the beginning of the central vowels. Classical singers, especially those employing the dropped mandible platform, are trained to create as much resonance and as much mouth aperture as possible so the richness of the phonemes can radiate into the atmosphere. However, the schwa is extremely difficult to produce in a mouth-open, dropped mandible platform state. The tongue profile quickly converts to either /ʌ/ or /ɛ/ if the mouth and mandible platform are too open.

Classical singers desiring to climb in the ranks must learn to use this vowel properly in its pure state if their diction is to be considered acceptable at the upper levels of the profession.

/ɚ/ Schwar—Mother. Much ink has been spilled over the ending -er sound in both English and German. One hears all kinds of solutions, the most common being the sub-stitution of /ʌ/ so that the word "moth*er*" is sung as /mʌðʌ/ instead of /mʌðɚ/. This is a classic case of creating one problem in an attempt to solve another, although as you will soon see, an understandable outcome.

The solution is the use of the legitimate phoneme, /ɚ/. Most writers about singing or acting would consider this to be a vowel plus a consonant. In doing so, one would need to choose from the various rhotic sounds (or "r-like" sounds) spanning from the trill /ř/ to the vocalic /ɐ/, and the uvular/guttural /r/ (more detail in Part II). Remember, the neutral vowel /ə/ is used for unstressed syllables, and both stressed /ɝ/ and unstressed /ɚ/ schwar are still containing part of it. For the schwar, however, looking at it as a single phoneme colored with a little /r/ (rhotic), in this case /ɐ/ (as in "father"—/fɑðɚ/), makes it a more authentic and proper solution to the -er problem. Thus, a "two-sound" phoneme is produced in which the first one is stronger, and the second one is weaker.

Doesn't that remind us of something? Yes, you guessed it right: pairs of vowels, in which one is the primary vowel (longer of the two) and the other the secondary vowel, are diphthongs. Therefore, the two sounds for our /ɚ/ are /ə/ + /ɐ/ = /əᵇ/ (Figure 6–13). (*Note:* in this book, we adopt the IPA system proposed by Garyth Nair in *The Craft of Singing* [2007], where we superscript the secondary vowel to make identification and performance easier.)

When singing or speaking a diphthong, the key is the distribution of the two different performance times (e.g., boy—/bɔ͡i/). The primary vowel has to be executed longer or otherwise we are turning it into a glide, /bᵓi/, where the secondary vowel is first (short), followed by a strong primary vowel (long) (e.g., want—/ʷʌnt/).

Are you beginning to see the predicament of our /ɚ/? The execution time—rapid passages versus long notes/emphasis—in singing and speaking of the schwar adds an additional challenge. Particularly, if one

has more time available, the /ə/ of our /əᵇ/ diphthong is often turned into a glide, leaving the majority of the remaining time for our secondary vowel /ɐ/, which most of the time results in the phonation of /ʌ/. *Et voilà*, now we have come full circle: put all elements—the tongue relaxation, too much mouth opening, and the lack of awareness—together and you will hear the /ʌ/ substitute for the /ɚ/ that singers/actors tend to produce and focus on.

Should you find yourself in the position that you do not have ample time for your diphthong, give the two vowels equal time. Under no circumstances should the secondary vowel of the diphthong ever receive the longer performance time. Because it is a diphthong and it is so open, the author suggests singers consider this as a legitimate vowel.

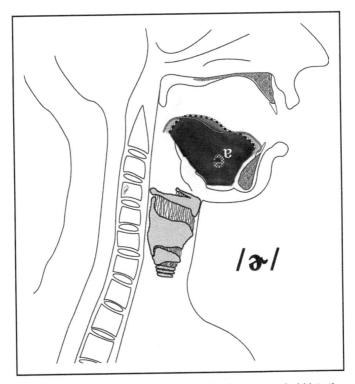

Figure 6–13. Overlay of the movement for the schwar /ɚ/. Note the subtle but effective change for the /r/ (*gray/checkered* or *yellow/red*) of the *-er*.

/ɝ/ Stressed Schwar—E<u>ar</u>th. It is the same with the *er-* found in the beginning (prefix) as well as *-er-* in midword position. The only difference is the starting position of our "two-sounds" phoneme, in this case the /ɜ/. As you can see in Figure 6–14, it is a bit farther back.

The desire, and properly so, is to avoid a hard (retroflex approximant, or tongue pulled too far back) /r/ (Figure 6–15).

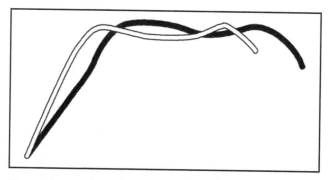

Figure 6–14. The central vowels /ɚ/ (schwar) in black/green, and the stressed schwar /ɝ/ in white/red.

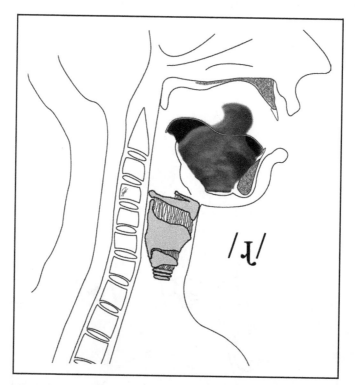

Figure 6–15. Retroflex /ɻ/ tongue shape. Note the extreme curled tongue tip (apex) creating a highly concave tongue shape. For comparison, the vocalic /r/ (/ɐ/), indicated by the tongue shape (*black/yellow*) and surface (*white/red*).

Unless, for instance, a singer in a musical or actor in a play needs to perform with a dialect, particularly one of the Midwestern United States.

However, as was the case with the word-final -er, substituting a non-schwa vowel is not a solution. Again, if the mouth is too open, a schwa converts into the vowel /ʌ/, and we hear /ʌθ/ instead of the idiomatic /ɝθ/.

The stressed schwar /ɝ/ is accomplished by pulling the tongue profile for the schwar slightly backward (see Figure 6–13). This imparts stronger rhotic timbre to the phoneme and results in the desired diction.

/æ/—That. The vowel /æ/ is a special case because some texts consider it a central vowel as it sits so and is relatively flat in the oral cavity (Figure 6–16).

Other vowels, such as /ɑ/, also sit low and seem to be almost similar in their 2D shape (see Figure 6–18, later in the chapter). So how is it that there is such a difference in not only vowel identification but also timbre? Since this question will reappear and concern us in the back vowels as well, we answer it then, though one clue is revealed right now: there is more "groove" in the tongue than one can see from the side.

/ʷ/ and /ʲ/—Two More Vowels You Thought Were Consonants

Similar to the /r/ in the er syllable, the letters /w/ and /y/ in English are considered consonants, though phonetically they are closer

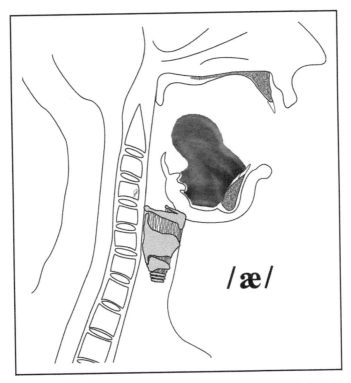

Figure 6–16. Tongue shape of the central phoneme /æ/, as in "th<u>a</u>t."

to vowel sounds, which is why in phonetics they are known as glides or semivowels. The IPA symbols for those phonemes are /ʷ/ and /ʲ/, and these speech sounds are related to the vowels /u/ (/ʷ/) and /i/ or /ɪ/ (/ʲ/).

Remember, we have just talked about the diphthong (see schwar above) and the importance of the distribution of the two different performance times of the primary vowel (longer) and secondary vowel (shorter). The contrary is true for glides.

They are like a "reversed diphthong" in that the secondary transitory vowel is executed first. Some examples of such glides are listed in Table 6–3.

In Figure 6–17, you see the tongue shape and movement for the glide /j/ derived from the ultrasound of the German word "*ja*" ("yes" in English). The movement is indicated by the two lines of which black/red is the starting point and white/green the end before changing to the vowel /ʌ/.

Table 6–3. Examples of /ʷ/ and /ʲ/ Glides in Various Languages

Glides	English	Italian	German	French
j	yes	iosa	ja	vien
w	wind	uomo		moi

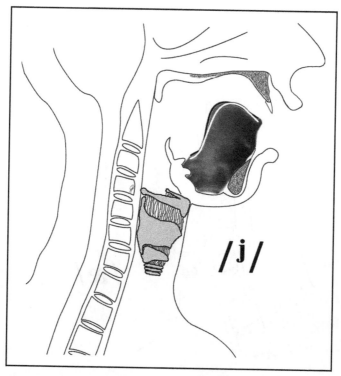

Figure 6–17. Tongue shape and movement (*indicated by the black/red and white/green lines*) of the glide /j/.

What is most striking about it is that the duration of the glide (from back/red to white/green) lasts only 0.06 sec or 60 msec, and the maximum distance is 4.7 mm (millimeters). To put it into perspective: the average duration for a single blink of a human eye is 0.1 to 0.4 sec, or 100 to 400 msec, according to the *Harvard Database of Useful Biological Numbers*. For purposes of comparison, the tick sound made by a clock lasts about 1 sec. So, it would be possible to either blink three times or make 17 glides during a single tick of a clock.

This example displays why the pronunciations of these secondary vowels are either massively exaggerated or substituted by other phonemes. Because they are shorter and transitory in nature, they do not leave much time to find either the right position or correction. Therefore, we need to know exactly the shape, position, and movement from start to finish before starting the process, or else we are not idiomatic in the language at hand and/or able to express, for instance, emotions without sounding ridiculous.

Back Vowels

Last but not least, to round up this chapter, we have back vowels. In a back vowel, the apex of the tongue is toward the bottom of the oral cavity. This creates a large space in the front of the oral cavity and a relatively smaller one in the back.

Remember our "two-rooms-connected-by-a-hallway" metaphor? The designations of our vowels (front, center, back) is based on *where* the tongue is when it divides the oral cavity in two. Until now, the tip (apex) of the tongue and the majority of its volume were in the front/center, creating a bigger resonance room in the back and

a smaller one in the front. The back vowels are the reverse. The tongue is moved back (and/or down) on the front (coronal) plane so that the larger resonance space is in the front.

The "*ah*" Variations

Our main goal in singing or acting is to pronounce the words properly for various reasons. First and foremost, of course, is to be idiomatic in any language or dialect, which in turn will ultimately result in an improvement of intelligibility. Second, depending on the contextual context or even lexical value (nouns, verbs versus pronouns and articles), we may want to somewhat exaggerate or modify the characteristics of the phoneme to get a point across. Third, we are continuously seeking variations in timbre in order to express different emotions. The latter is of particular importance for consonants, because I am not only advocating consonant resonance (CR; Chapter 7) for intelligibility but also strongly believe that consonants carry the majority of the emotions we aspire to convey (Chapter 1).

As you can see, Figure 6–18 shows various "a" vowels. Remember the vowel /æ/? In the same way as we saw in our central vowel, it also sits low and relatively flat in the oral cavity. So why is there such a difference in not only vowel identification but also timbre?

The "Groove"

To look further into the question posed, we have to first remind ourselves of the hydrostatic nature of the tongue. In other words, no matter how we change the structure/shape of the tongue, it always preserves its volume (see Chapter 3). For example, when

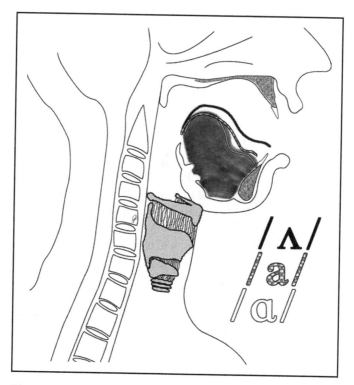

Figure 6–18. Contours of various "a" vowels, concluding with the actual tongue shape of /ɑ/. Note the changes in the concavity and waveform of the tongue surface, starting from moderate in /ʌ/ to more pronounced in /ɑ/.

you see a compression in the front (anterior) of the tongue as in Figure 6–19, it will be compensated by an expansion of the back (posterior) of the tongue. Hence, the shape of the tongue is "volume-preserving," so that every local compression is compensated for by an expansion. Think of a water balloon, no matter how you squeeze it, it will bulge in order to preserve the volume.

Looking again at Figure 6–18, you can see that all three phonemes have a similar 2D shape in the form of a wave. However, the moderate concavity in /ʌ/ progressively increases for /a/ and /ɑ/, gradually compressing the front of the tongue downward while increasingly protruding the back. Whereas these minimal changes already have a huge acoustic impact (see reflection Chapter 3),

wait until you see what happens in addition to that when we look at the tongue from the front (coronal). We are going to somewhat mimic a 3D perspective in stages by turning the transducer 90°, which changes the perspective from the side (sagittal), as in Figure 6–18, to the front (coronal), as in Figure 6–19. Remember the big, fan-shaped muscle (Chapter 2, Figure 2–7) called the genioglossus (GG)? This muscle, circled with a dotted/yellow oval in the left image in Figure 6–19, depresses the tongue, creating a little "groove" (indicated by the arrow). The same can be observed in the ultrasound image on the right.

If we overlay the groove contours of each vowel (Figure 6–20), we observe the same gradual increase of concavity from

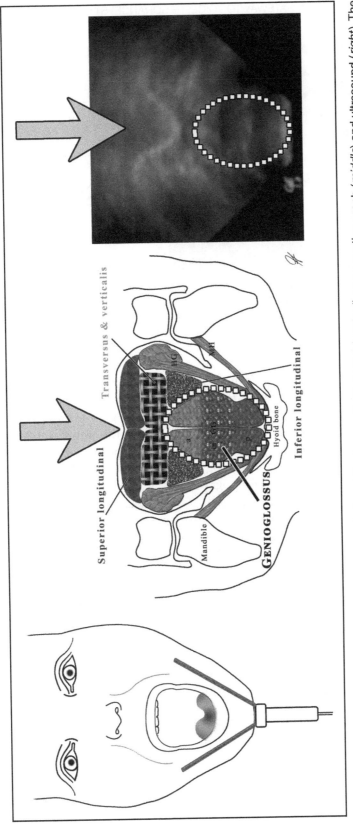

Figure 6–19. Transducer turned 90° for a front (anterior) view of the tongue (*left*), frontal (coronal) cross-section graph (*middle*) and ultrasound (*right*). The genioglossus depresses (*dotted/yellow oval*), creating the "groove" (*indicated by the arrow*).

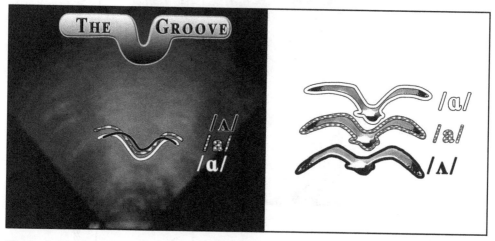

Figure 6–20. Front view of an overlay of various "a" vowels contours, concluding with the ultrasound image (*left*) of the actual tongue contour of /ɑ/. Note the increase in the groove depth of the tongue surface, starting from moderate in /ʌ/ to a more pronounced one in /ɑ/. Fascinatingly enough, the contours closely resemble the wing flaps of a bird (*right*).

/ʌ, a, to ɑ/. Only now the wave is more of a groove along the midline of the tongue whose depth increases.

We can also see the shift on the spectrogram by using the power spectrum. As mentioned in Chapter 5, voice pedagogy already uses virtual real-time spectrography for eye-body biofeedback. Garyth Nair, in his book *Voice-Tradition and Technology* (1999), already illustrated how computer feedback can service to find those various norms. Like the power spectrum, Figure 6–21 shows the formant pattern for these vowels obtained by using Donald Miller's "vocal fry" method (where the vocal folds compress rather tightly and become relatively slack and compact, thus virtually eliminating the harmonics and leaving only format producing resonance of the vocal tract). You can see how the first two formants (indicated by the arrows) shifted to the right (higher frequency) for the /ʌ/ vowel (as in m<u>o</u>ther). Also of note is the on average greater intensity (level) shown in the midsection of the spectrum.

Now, have a look again at Figure 6–6 at the beginning of this chapter. Can you see the various grooves along the A-axes? For /i/ and /e/, the groove is more in the back (posterior) portion of the tongue, while the front (anterior) reaches the upper border of axis A. Moving along, it turns into a more continuous midline groove in /ɪ/ and continues to increase the depth along the entire tongue in /ɛ/ and /æ/. With the ultrasound, we can move the transducer to follow the groove and make sure, for instance, we have it in the back of the tongue for the vowel /i/ (Figure 6–22). But the indications of a groove can also be observed from a side (sagittal) perspective. Looking at Figure 6–23, you will see that the presence or absence of a groove is clearly recognizable as either a hump (no groove) or dimple (groove).

Since one of the key elements in consonants is to maintain high-frequencies turbulence associated with, for example, fricatives such as /ʃ/ (as in "<u>sh</u>ow"), the groove will be of particular importance for us when we deal with consonant resonance (CR).

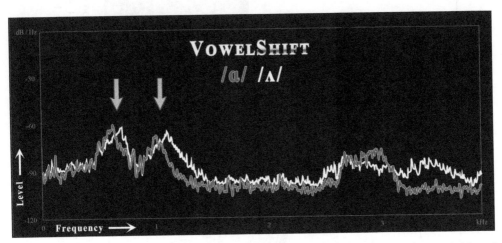

Figure 6–21. A power spectrum showing the formants (*yellow arrows*) of the sung /ɑ/ (*gray/green*) and /ʌ/ (*white/red*).

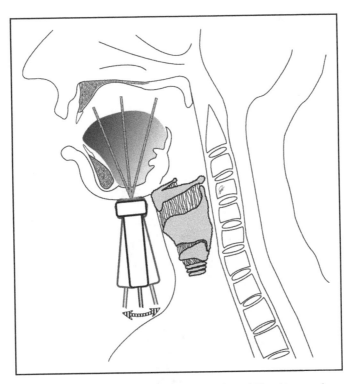

Figure 6–22. Moving transducer along the midline (A-axes from Figure 6–6) to watch the groove in the front, middle, or back of the tongue.

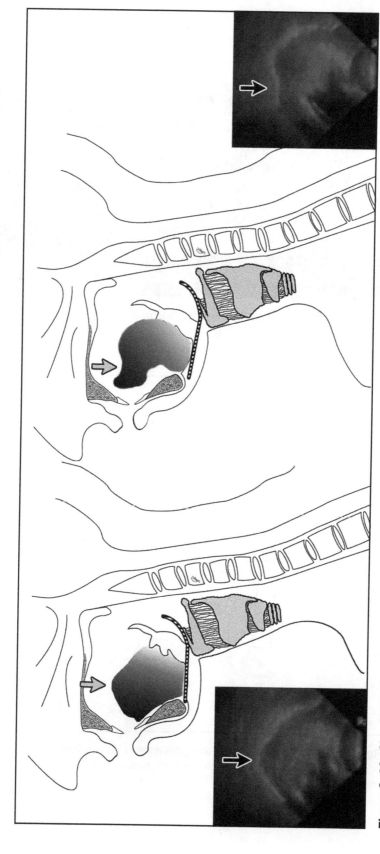

Figure 6–23. Side (sagittal) profile of the consonant /ʃ/ (*show*) without consonant resonance (*left*) and with consonant resonance (*right*), accompanied by their original ultrasound images. The hump on the left indicates that there is no groove in the front of the tongue, whereas the dimple on the right implies that a groove is present. Also, note the change in the jaw (mandible) line (*striped/red*). For the groove, it drops in the back (posterior) in order to maintain the lower frequencies as well (Chapter 7).

More on that exciting subject is presented in Chapter 7 and Part II.

Now that we have found "the groove" in our tongue, we can fully answer our question of why there is such a difference in both vowel identification and timbre, even though the various "a" vowels in Figure 6–18 or even our central vowel /æ/ (Figure 6–16) have a similar 2D shape in the form of a wave. So, if a singer or actor sings/speaks a proper /ɑ/ (as in "law," or the German "Wagen"), the tongue is at its farthest configuration from its at-rest position (deeper concavity in the front and more mass in the back). However, if that full concavity of the /ɑ/ is not diligently maintained, the tongue will relax, and the phoneme will drift toward either the /a/ or /ʌ/ vowels, changing the 2D wave shape as well as the 3D shape, such as the groove depth (see Figures 6–18 and 6–20). Concomitant to the physiological change of the entire tongue shape, we have, according to the source-filter theory (Chapter 5), a change in filter, and consequently the formants (see Figure 6–21).

/o/, /ɔ/, /u/, /ʊ/—Motor (German), ox, moon, put

Continuing on our vowel journey, we have a few more back vowels before we can round up this chapter. Please note that I am using the German "Motor" instead of the English "motor" for the phoneme /o/. Unfortunately, I was not able to find an English example where the single phoneme /o/ does not turn into a diphthong. The primary vowel of the diphthong (see Chapter 5) in the word "pope" may be the closest to the single /o/.

With some of the main indicators introduced, I am sure you can already analyze and interpret the differences of the various tongue shapes. Let us start with the phoneme pair /o/ (Motor) and /ɔ/ (ox) in Figure 6–24. Their 2D shape is obviously different. Both have a wave shape, although different in their extent, compressing the tip (apex) of the tongue (indicative for the groove in the front because of a depressed genioglossus muscle).

What is interesting in this case is the almost disappearing divide of our "two-room-hallway" (Chapter 5) in the phoneme /o/. The back of the tongue does not protrude as much as in /ɔ/, and the "hump" itself looks even smaller. Again, think 3D and remember the hydrostatic (volume preserving) nature of the tongue. This means that the mass of the back of the tongue has to move somewhere else because—yes, you guessed it—we also have a little bit of a groove in the back of the tongue that pushes the remaining mass to the side.[2] As a result, it almost depresses the entire tongue downward (as if you would sit on it) and opens up the divide of the oral (mouth) and pharyngeal (throat) cavity.

The 2D modifications concerning our other phoneme pair /u/ (moon) and /ʊ/ (put) are prominent as well (Figure 6–25).

Similar indicators as in /o/ and /ɔ/ can be observed. Only now a more noticeable divide of our "two-room-hallway" is evident because the depression of the back of the tongue is not present. What does stand out is the similarity of the two open phonemes /ɔ/ and /ʊ/. In an overlay of those phonemes (Figure 6–26), one can see that this is not the case at all. From the side (sagittal), you can see differences in the degree of concavity, the overall form of the wave shape, and the position of the tongue. Turning 90° to the front (coronal), the difference in concavity and depth of their groove become apparent (see Figure 6–26).

---

[2]Three-dimensional imaging from Stone and Lundberg, A. (1996) as well as front (coronal) ultrasound scans confirm the existence of the groove in the back.

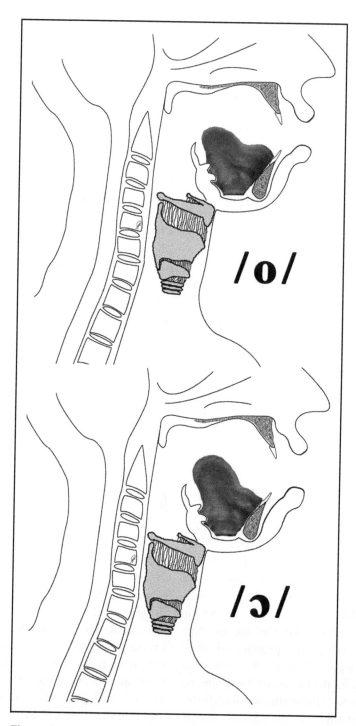

Figure 6–24. Tongue shapes of the phonemes /o/ (m<u>o</u>tor) and /ɔ/ (<u>o</u>x).

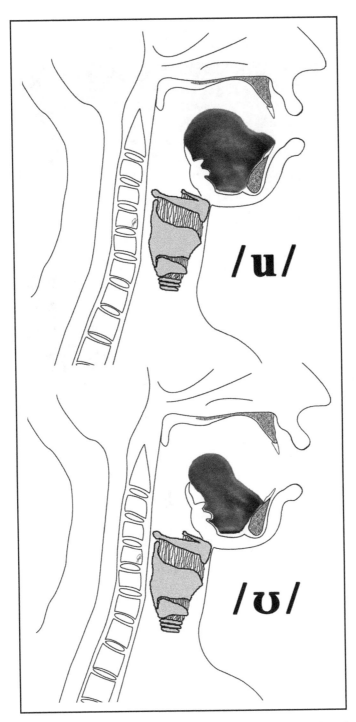

Figure 6–25. Tongue shapes of the phonemes /u/ (moon) and /ʊ/ (put).

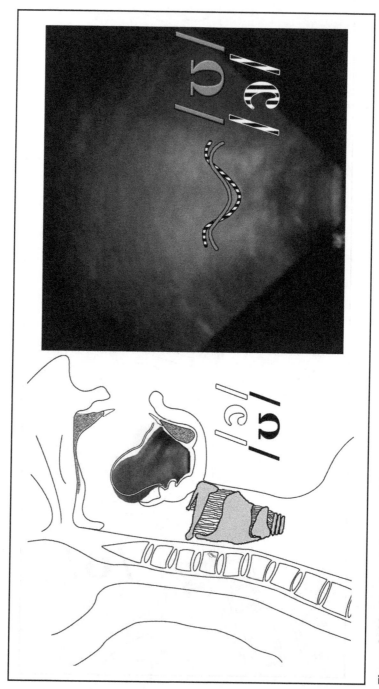

Figure 6–26. Overlay of phonemes /ɔ/ and /ʊ/ from the side (sagittal, *left*) and the front (coronal, *right*).

Now that we have tackled these important basic aspects of the tongue physiology and their concomitant acoustic changes, we have set the basis for the central subject of this book: consonant resonance. With this understanding of how great singing or SAS vowels with good resonance work, our consonants resonance parity with our vowels can be achieved. So, let us finally dive into the fascinating world of consonants.

References

Lee, S. H., Kwon, H. J., Choi, H. J., Lee, N. H., Lee, S. J., & Jin, S. M. (2008). The singer's formant and speaker's ring resonance: A long-term average spectrum analysis. *Clinical and Experimental Otorhinolaryngology, 1*(2), 92–96. https://doi.org/10.3342/ceo.2008.1.2.92

Nair, G. (2007). *The craft of singing.* San Diego, CA: Plural Publishing.

Nair, A., Nair, G., & Reishofer, G. (2016). The low mandible maneuver and its resonential implications for elite singers. *Journal of Voice, 30,* 128.e13–128.e32

Stone, M. (1990). A three-dimensional model of tongue movement based on ultrasound and x-ray microbeam data. *Journal of the Acoustical Society of America, 87*(5), 2207–2217.

Stone, M., & Lundberg, A. (1996). Three-dimensional tongue surface shapes of English consonants and vowels. *Journal of the Acoustical Society of America, 99*(6), 3728–3737.

7 Consonants and Consonant Resonance

In Chapter 1, it was shown that the main reason for this almost ancient struggle with consonants is that the rapidity of their execution leaves no time to focus on their production. As a result, most singers and actors sing/recite with considerably improved vowels interspersed with ineffective consonants. So, let us get our phonetician's head on and have a thorough look into what consonants actually are in order to learn to consciously apply and manipulate their production.

One could oversimplify and say that consonants are any phonemes that are not vowels. You will soon see, however, that this is in fact a great way to classify consonants, because of the wide variations in their production. We already classified the vowels—one of the two types of phonemes (a single language sound, see Chapter 5)—as a sound produced by a vocal tract that is more or less unobstructed; thus, it is a sound that is produced by an open vocal tract. Consonants, on the other hand, result from a **degree of obstruction/constriction**. The many variations of obstruction can range from

- *a complete closure of the vocal tract,* in which the airflow out of the mouth is completely stopped, to
- *a partial closure of the vocal tract,* where some airflow is permitted to pass and exit, and is accompanied by a degree of turbulence or friction-like noise.

The task of classifying speech sounds in general is by no means trivial. We therefore focus on what are, for us, the most eminent concerns.

Voicing: Pitch-Nonpitch (Consovowels-Consonants)

This book is focused on the performance of well-sung or "say it as a singer" (SAS) phonemes and not solely theoretical classifications or techniques of printed/spoken languages. This is why we start with the consonant division of

- *pitch* (those that involve phonation at the vocal folds) and
- *nonpitch* (those that have no element of phonation → noise).

The distinction of the two is of particular importance to a performer because anything that includes pitch adds an additional layer of considerations regarding the physiological setup and its acoustic ramifications. But let us not jump ahead; let us define the classification in more detail first.

I. Voicing: Pitch Versus Nonpitch,
II. Place of Articulation, and
III. Manner of Articulation.

Pitch (Consovowels)

We adopt the classification by Garyth Nair (2007), who classifies *any* consonant that can be *sustained on pitch* as a ***consovowel*** (consonant + vowel). Nair expanded the term—originally coined by Henderson and Palmer (1940) and covering only the phonemes /m, n, ŋ, l, and r/—to include all consonants executed on pitch. He also showed spectrographic evidence in which these consonants show a "vowel-like harmonic development." (*Note:* in phonetics and phonology, you may read the terms *voiced/voicing* or *unvoiced/voiceless* to characterize the same distinction of consonants.)

Remember what we can see on a spectrogram (Chapter 1)? Have a look at Figure 7–1 where you can see wave lines stacked above each other. These are the individual harmonics (i.e., the **fundamental tone** $[f_o]$ plus its various **overtones** $[1f_o, 2f_o, 3f_o,$ etc., above it] that appear when an instrument, such as the human voice through vocal folds, vibrates [oscillates]). Please note that in this book, we adapt the old notation of **harmonics** (H_1, H_2,

H_3, etc.) to the new one, introduced in the consensus document by Titze et al. (2015).

In Figure 7–2, the vocal folds are shown from a bird's-eye view, similar to that which an otolaryngologist (ENT) or speech pathologist would see when using a laryngostroboscope (a flexible or rigid instrument with a light source and camera that is inserted, respectively, through the nose or mouth and enables the user to view and record laryngeal function in real time).

When we breathe, our vocal folds are in an at-rest position and look, interestingly enough, like a "V" as in "voice" (Figure 7–2, left). Overly simplified, this means that they are apart from each other (**abducted**) when we breathe and come together (**adducted**) in rapid wave motions (hundreds of times per second) modulating the flow of air being expelled from the lungs during phonation (Figure 7–2, right) (see Nair, 2007; Sataloff, 2005; Sundberg, 1987; Titze, 2000). The latter shows up on the spectrogram as harmonics (see Figure 7–1).

What does that look like in terms of Garyth Nair's spectrographic evidence of

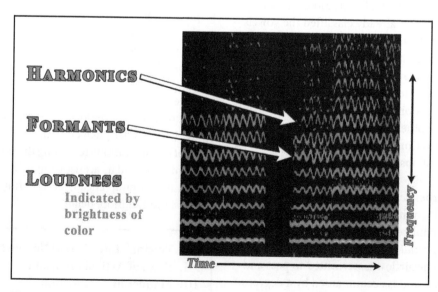

Figure 7–1. What we can see from a spectrogram of sung phonemes.

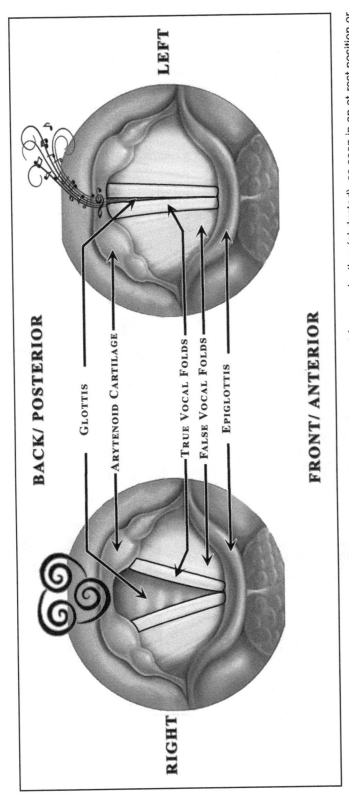

Figure 7–2. Vocal folds viewed from above look like a "V." On the left, they are apart from each other (abducted), as seen in an at-rest position or when breathing; thus, only air is coming through. On the right, the folds are together (adducted) and (under the right conditions) create sounds that, on the spectrograph, would appear as harmonics.

consovowels (all consonants with pitch)? When you look at Figure 7–3, you can see how every one of these consonants displays vowel-like harmonics, which is why we need to pay special attention to them. Intonation and volume of consovowels greatly enhance the recitation/song or keep, for example, essential criteria such as vocal line, richness in sound, and intelligibility. Just think about what all you can do with an "m" in the word /mʌin/ ("mine"). Start the recitation with a higher pitch on the "m" and you get more desperation, or sustain and slowly increase the volume on a medium pitch and you stretch the "mhhhomentum." As discussed in Chapter 1, consonants carry much (if not most) of the burden of dramatic interpretation in singing and acting. The consovowels here offer an almost infinite color palette of emotions, and this kind of attention to detail not only puts the work of an artist into a professional rank but makes it truly exciting.

Singers are faced with an additional challenge when singing the consovowels. Because of the pitch component, one has to sing them on the actual pitch of the immediately following vowel that it is paired with. When a singer begins the pitch consonant even just slightly below this pitch, it will result in the technical fault we all know as

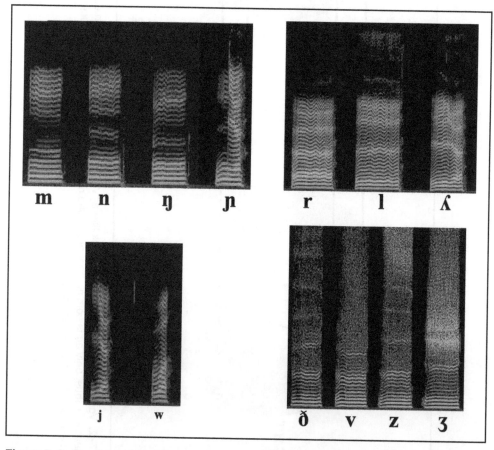

Figure 7–3. Spectrograms of the consovowels showing the vowel-like harmonic development stemming from the vibration of the vocal folds. From *The Craft of Singing* (p. 305) by Garyth Nair. Copyright © 2007 Plural Publishing, Inc. All Rights Reserved.

"scooping" (Figure 7–4). Unless a certain vocal style requires a specific and consciously/purposely applied scoop, which also has to start on a certain pitch for timing and effect, otherwise it will affect both sound and style; this is certainly not a desirable result and can often turn into a somewhat annoying affectation. More often than not, the incentive to the singer—that the scoop habituates itself—is because it either "feels" emotional and personally satisfying and/or compensates a lack of technique (not having enough airflow, etc.). In Figure 7–4, you can observe that in the scoop,

- the harmonics are rising until they arrive at the actual pitch (440 Hz),

- the transition from the consovowel /m/ to the vowel /a/ is rough, and
- the misalignment continues into the vowel (waves are not steady).

On the other hand, the on-pitch /m/ shows

- an alignment of the harmonics from the very start of the /m/ to the end of the secondary vowel of the diphthong /i/,
- a smooth transition from the consovowel /m/ to the vowel /a/, and
- the vowel is not affected by any disturbance.

Because of the vowel component in our consovowels, singers also have to pay

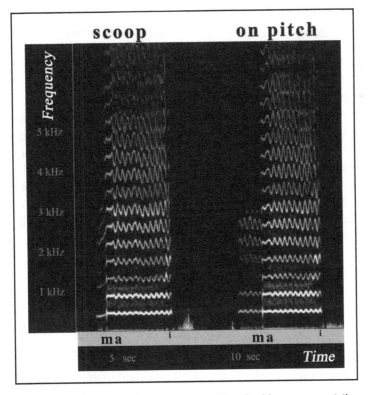

Figure 7–4. Spectrogram of the word "my" with a scoop at the beginning of the /m/ on the left and a properly, on-pitch, performed /m/ on the right. Also, note the cleaner and smoother transition from the consovowels /m/ to the vowel /a/ in the on-pitch version.

attention to modifying them as well when they approach their *passaggi* (Italian for "passages" from one register to another). This process of vowel modification (blending areas of the voice quality into a timbral continuum) is very complicated, though a critical part in our quest for well-executed consonants. It requires a look into some numbers. However, bear with me on that one because the following will be a gross simplification on what vowel **modification** (or formant tuning) is in order to obtain an understanding of the concept. There is much more to it than what you are about to read, which is why I strongly recommend—particularly for voice pedagogues/practitioners—consulting Miller (2008), Nair (2007), Sundberg (1987), and Titze (2000) for more details on both *passaggi* and vowel modification.

Vowel Modification

What is **vowel modification?** To answer this rather complex question, let us first remind ourselves and put together a few puzzle pieces, beginning with resonance (Figure 7–5). Remember, in Chapter 3 we looked at the semioccluded vocal tract (SOVT) or semienclosed airspace. We all have our own personal dimensions and shapes of our vocal tract; thus, we have a certain resonant frequency determined by the various parameters (length, diameters, volumes, etc.) (Chapter 5). This is why two women singing the same pitch and vowel have a different sound. In Chapter 5, we used the analogy of blowing across a bottle's top, showing how that creates its own resonant frequency (formants). Similar to a person who has an identity document (ID) that proves that person's identity, so has our vocal tract a specific ID, only now we call it resonant frequency (formants) instead of date of birth, retina, fingerprints, and so on. However, unlike a fingerprint, we are able

to manipulate our parameters of the vocal tract by changing the shape and concomitant diameter, length, and so on, with our active articulators, such as the tongue. This enables us, for instance, to create various vowel sounds and timbres (Chapter 5, formants, source-filter theory).

Another puzzle piece is the pitch frequency. In the spectrograph, we already saw the stack of wave lines of which the lowest is the ID of the fundamental frequency (f_0), which is the actual pitch we hear (e.g., 440 Hz for middle A_4). All others above represent the individual harmonics of the fundamental (also sometimes referred to as **partials** or overtones), which the human ear does not perceive as separate phenomena.

Both frequencies, the resonant frequency of the vocal tract and the pitch frequency, are now meeting within the vocal tract. As discussed in Chapter 5, some areas in the vocal tract like to boost certain harmonics. This is always a challenging subject—particularly in the pedagogical domain—that is hard at first for both young teachers and students to conceptualize, visualize, or comprehend for that matter. This is why I would like to offer the following experiment that may arguably be farfetched; however, it empirically proves to be helpful in the understanding of the concept and tactile experience of this "frequency meeting."

Exercise—"Frequency Meeting"

Before you execute the experiment, explain the following steps to your student so he or she knows what to expect:

1. Ask the student to sing and sustain on a comfortable, open (relaxed jaw), and supported (engaged lower abdominal muscles) pitch.
2. The teacher joins by singing a half-step higher than the student's chosen

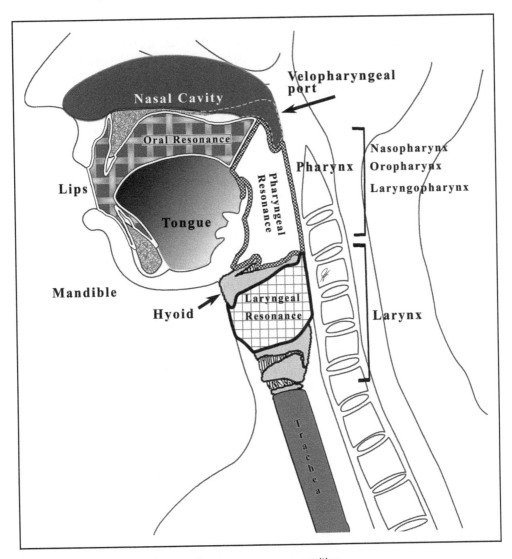

Figure 7–5. Sagittal (side) view of various resonance cavities.

pitch in close proximity of each other (almost face-to-face).

3. Try to avoid the temptation to adjust and resolve the beautiful dissonance.

4. While singing, take in both tactile (anywhere, e.g., mouth, facial skin, etc.) and auditive sensations. Repeat the exercise a couple of times since it can be hard for some to either maintain the pitch or are just irritated by the instable sound or tactile sensations.

5. Next, repeat the experiment but now the teacher matches the student's pitch. Again, take in the various sensations (tactile, auditive, etc.) and then compare the two.

The first one feels very unstable because the harmonic(s) (the stacked wave lines) of the half-step higher tone sung by the teacher do not perfectly/exactly line up with the harmonics of the original lower frequency tone sung by the student. This not only expresses itself in a much more brain-intensive and difficult perception of the sound but also in the increased vibration perceived on the facial skin. One can feel the collision and bouncing of the non-matching wave lines. However, when it is a match—in other words, both singing the same pitch, thus the harmonics line up and coincide with each other—it is not only a more pleasurable, resolving perception but also reinforced, boosted/amplified sound (see Chapters 3 and 5).

Now, with those experiences in mind, slowly sing a little scale or phrase over a wider span, possibly along one of the transition zones (*passaggi*), and observe within the vocal tract if there are moments that may feel unstable, like in the experiment. If so, we likely need to modify. This, of course, is particularly true in the areas of the transitions (first passaggio between D_4–F_4, second passaggio between D_5–F_5). Why and what is that? Well, there are a multitude of reasons that can occur on an anatomical/physiological (laryngeal muscular adjustment) or acoustic (resonance tuning) level. Since we have been talking about vocal tract frequency and pitch frequency, we are—you may have already guessed—going to be focusing on the acoustic part. However, as you will soon see, it involves another muscular adjustment: the reshaping of the tongue.

So, let us talk about that always dreaded transition. The vowels have a specific "frequency constellation" or better "vocal tract resonance" (see Chapter 5) that allows us to perceive and identify them as "a, e, i, o, *or* u." Only now, as discussed earlier, we call them formant frequencies and label them Formant 1 and 2 (F_1, F_2; see Chapters 3 and 5). On the left in Figure 7–6 you see a vowel chart (after Peterson & Barney, 1952) showing the constellation F_1, F_2 for each vowel (e.g., /ɪ/ → F_1 = ~430; F_2 = ~2700). (*Note*: these are approximate numbers that descend for males' and ascend for females' or children's voices due to the different sizes of the vocal tract [see Chapters 3 and 5].)

Now, we are going to look at these two IDs (pitch and vowel) to see how they can correspond or compete with each other, especially when we sing in the areas where we move from one register to another (*passaggi*). Let us assume that we sing a scale, starting at middle A_4 and going up to A_5. Naturally, we can hear the pitch raising, which means that the f_o of 440 Hz (which is A_4) rises to 880 Hz (= A_5), as indicated by the vertical lines in Figure 7–6. So far so good. If we want to sing that scale on the vowel /ɪ/ (as in "p<u>i</u>n"), the F_1 = ~430 Hz is just slightly below though still in close vicinity of our f_o of 440 Hz (pitch A_4) we start our scale with. However, if we keep ascending in our scale, you can see that f_o is moving away from that F_1 frequency, essentially exceeding it. Take a pencil or so, align it with the vertical line of A_4, and move it to the right to picture it. If we maintain the F_1 of our /ɪ/ while raising our pitch (which means we are not changing anything in the shape of our vocal tract set for the vowel), the acoustic result is not pleasant. The intonation of the pitch is often flat, the sound is pushed, and the larynx feels tight, or worse, hurts. This is because our raising f_o is "held back" by the F_1, not allowing it to move freely without losing its integrity (remember, right now we are only focusing on the acoustic part, not the anatomical/physiological adjustment that also plays a role in it).

Exercise—"Frequency Meeting" Visualization

Let us try to visualize that with our hands (Figure 7–7): the left hand represents the F_1 of the vowel, and the right hand is the f_o of

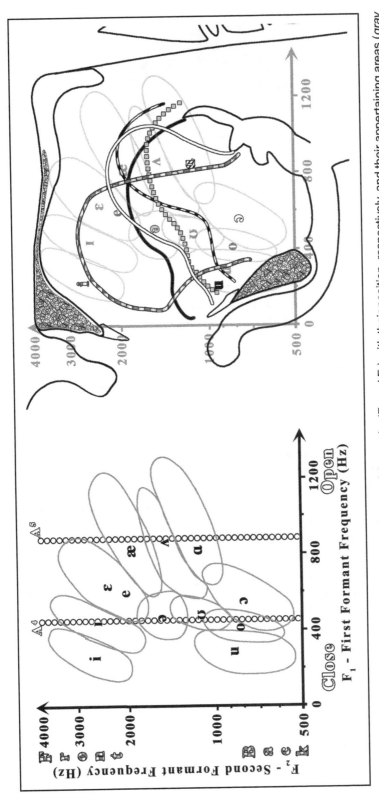

Figure 7–6. *Left:* Vowel chart indicating the frequencies of the peaks (F$_1$ and F$_2$) with their position, respectively, and their appertaining areas (*gray circle*) due to variations in articulative configurations and vocal tract size. The pitches (A4 and A5) are marked by the vertical lines (*dotted/bright green*). *Right:* An approximate overlay of the vowel chart with some vowel tongue shapes. Note how the various shapes influence the shift of F$_1$ and F$_2$.

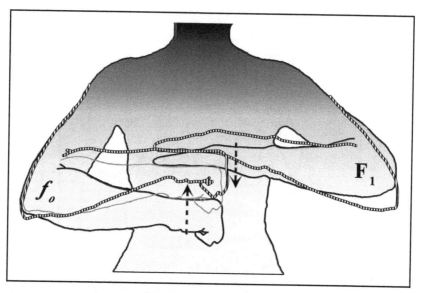

Figure 7–7. The hand on the left mimics the raising pitch (f_o) of the scale, while the hand on the right (F1) prevents it from continuing, by pushing down.

the pitch. Move the left hand, palm down, in front of you and maintain it leveled at the end of your lower rib cage (or another fixed position). Now, make a fist with your right hand, and position it below your left hand. Remember to keep your left hand leveled at set position. Next, begin to move the right hand up (as you would sing the scale). Once you hit your left hand, your right hand wants to push through your left hand. However, your left hand is preventing your right hand from continuing freely because it keeps pushing it down. You may force your way through it, though that "fight" does not feel good in either hand (remember the fight of our dissonances).

You may ask now, what can we do to avoid this physically and acoustically rather unpleasant event? We need to make sure that f_o does not exceed F_1. How? By finding a vowel whose F_1 does not exceed or stays within close proximity to f_o when ascending the pitch up to the 800-Hz mark. Did you find it in Figure 7–6? Yes, /ʌ/, ɑ, and æ/ look

like good candidates for this *vowel modification* because their F_1 is around the 800-Hz mark. So, instead of stubbornly maintaining the /ɪ/ throughout the scale (which is because of our speech template, Chapter 1), we *modify* (not change) the pharyngeal area (Chapter 3) with one of the following three phonemes: /ʌ/, ɑ, and æ/. In other words, while setting the tongue for the vowel /ɪ/, we simultaneously mold /ʌ/, ɑ, or æ/ into the shape (like a merger) that changes the space in the back of the mouth (pharyngeal area). Have a look now at the right image of Figure 7–6, to compare the tongue shapes for /i/ and /ɑ/. Can you see the difference? Again, at first, we are not changing the entire tongue into the /ɑ/ shape (except for the sky-high coloratura part . . . there we only make it work with the best vowel possible). At the beginning of the scale, imagine keeping the vertical integrity of the /ɪ/ shape in the front of the surface of the tongue, but mold everything underneath (body/root part, see Part II) into an /ɑ/. Moving up the scale, you increase this molding more and more, which, of course, will jeopardize the vowel intelligibility, though if done continuously and gradually, we are keeping the illusion of the vowel /ɪ/ alive. Current ultrasound research of the tongue morphology in vowel modification conducted by the author shows evidence of exactly that and also how the modifying (molding) part eventually turns into a complete transformation of the vowel (more on that in another paper and book).

Now you may wonder, why isn't /ʌ/ the winner, since it is the closest to the 800-Hz mark? We are individuals (different sizes of vocal tract: e.g., male versus female), and there are many more aspects that have to be considered in this process (e.g., articulative configuration, etc.). Thus, every singer has to find the modifier best suitable for their instrument in order to guarantee an open, free, in-tune, and intelligable sound throughout the scale. Ideally, you set up a **formant profile** (similar to a voice profile [Titze & Verdolini, 2000]), where you find your personal formants for each vowel, so you know exactly how to modify for both your passaggi (register transitions) and your timbral output.

Before we continue to dicuss the former in the context of consovowels, here is a quick note regarding timbre: it is very easy to forget that we need to find not only the ideal modifier vowel but also the vowel that helps us filter out those harmonics (stack of waves) that will give us the desired timbre (e.g., brassy, dark, etc.). Keep in mind that perception is an important puzzle piece in the orchestration of vocal quality, or sometimes also described by the term *register*. By filtering different harmonics, we can change the vowel or its acoustic properties. For instance, more often than not, the intuitive reaction of a singer or actor is to change the source (vocal folds) by increasing the vocal effort (e.g., pushing harder through extra laryngeal muscles tension or the like) to accomplish either more intensity (loudness), brassiness in the sound, and/or avoid instabilities because the decoupling of source and filter (vocal tract) is not yet established. This is why—besides laryngeal position, lip formation, and jaw position—the tongue is a crucial part in terms of source-filter interaction (Chapter 5). So when one finds certain instabilities or wants to change voice qualities for stylistic, dynamic, and/or aesthetic reasons, we can reshape and change the vocal tract with our active articulators, particularly the tongue.

The tongue and by extension its concommitant meticulous work through the lens of tongue morphology that goes into vocal production in general as well as vowel modification is a significant puzzle piece that has not yet been explicitly addressed and is often overlooked, neglected, or even avoided. While this book aims to help change this status quo, I would like to reiterate that given the complex nature of vocal production, it is not the only one.

Exercise—Consovowel Modification

Let us continue and translate all of this into our sung *consovowels* and reveal an aspect of consonant production that is too often neglected by practitioners and singers alike. We have just seen that consovowels contain vowel-like harmonics and thus are sung on a pitch. This means that the *same rules of vowel modification* have to be applied when we reach the areas of register change (*passaggi*). The vowel behind the consonant is the one immediately following it. For instance, in /mi/, the /m/ would be sung with the resonance of /i/ (as in "keen") behind it. Thus, when singing a five-note-scale on /m/ and on top of the scale opening up to the vowel /i/, we have to also make sure to modify the /m/ accordingly. Assuming, if I, a mezzo/contralto, would sing the scale, I would use the modifier /ɑ/ (which works best for me) immediately from the beginning, so I would not only maintain a well-sung /m/ but also be ready and set for the approaching /i/ vowel (Figure 7–8, top). This is also a good exercise for proper consovowel production.

Of course, one is probably more likely to find something like on the bottom of Figure 7–8, although some avant-garde music can require unconventional methods of syllabic execution. Anyway, in this example you want to start singing the consovowel on the pitch E$_5$ and also modify it with the modifier that you will be using for the /i/ vowel. Otherwise, if the consovowel is not modified, one will not only lose their sound, resonance, and intonation in the consonant, but consequently, the vowel will suffer as well (Figure 7–4; Chapter 1). In Part II of the book, some of the pitfalls on each consovowel and tongue positions are listed in more detail.

Consonant Resonance

Having gone through the classification of consovowels (pitch, voiced consonants) and the consequential necessary modification of their vowel-like part, you can see why we had to first establish the phonetics and resonance from a vowel perspective. Because with the understanding of how great sung or SAS vowels work (Chapter 5), we are now able to grant the consonants resonential parity with our vowels. This is why it is time to introduce the term that is specific to that concept and that has already been referred to throughout this book, in more detail: **consonant resonance (CR)**. Originally the term and concept were introduced by Garyth Nair (1999) to remind the singer to continually regard the potential gain in resonance for the production of *all* consonants. With the ultrasound as an additional research and biofeedback tool, the author further examines that "secret" and is able to confirm and add to the findings of Garyth Nair.

Remember how the movable parts (articulators, e.g., tongue, lips, jaw, etc.) in our vocal tract filter the source (sound), changing the reflection and thus the for-

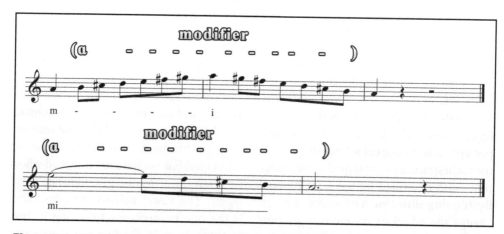

Figure 7–8. Five-note-scales from A4 (440 Hz) to E5 (659 Hz) on /mi/ with the modifier /ɑ/ (for the author's voice) indicated above (*gray/green*). *Top:* Starting the scale with /m/ and opening up to /i/ on the top note. *Bottom:* Start again with /m/, then on the second beat open up to /i/.

mants (IDs) of our phonemes (Chapter 5). We also looked at the tongue from both a two-dimensional (2D) and three-dimensional (3D) perspective, pointing out various tongue shape indications for each vowel, and "the groove" was of particular interest (Chapter 5). We continue from there, though now examine its importance for our consonants.

So far, we have seen that the tongue with its intrinsic and extrinsic muscles is one of the most malleable articulators, shaping itself into the most remarkable shapes while keeping its volume (hydrostat). Most vowels showed a distinctive 2D shape, yet some exhibited close similarities. But on a closer look, we found the "groove" with its various concavities (Figure 7–9).

How do those changes affect our consonants? For our consovowels, the answer may seem almost too obvious or even primitive. Since their resonance is mainly established through the immediately following vowel, we just need to make sure to set the tongue accordingly. Let us look at an example where we sing a sequence of a vowel and consovowel (e.g., /amama/). Although it does not carry as much upper-harmonic development, the spectrographic image in Figure 7–10 shows how easily the /m/ blends with the vowel when sung with CR. And, since this book proposes the same setup for an actor's well-projected spoken voice, we also compare a SAS and regular spoken sequence that also show a clear difference in harmonics for both vowel and consovowel. Why is the /m/ in general so poor in harmonic richness? Because of the mouth closure, the uvula (nasopharyngeal port) has to open in order to redirect the airflow and sound through the nose. As a result, a significant dampening of the higher frequencies occurs, thus taking away acoustic power. We ought to keep in mind the two-chamber hallway metaphor (Chapter 5).

Their volume is determined by the tongue shape and position of the tongue. Because of the mouth closure, the oral cavity becomes a side chamber to this pathway. This is why we need to pay attention to it, because theoretical and empirical studies of the spectral properties of nasals indicate that this side chamber can contribute to antiresonances (Fant, 1960; Fujimura, 1962; Ladefoged & Maddieson, 1996; Recasens, 1983).

This makes it all the more necessary to utilize the full potential of CR for both sung and SAS consovowels. Otherwise, we lose the balance between vowel and consonant, and as we saw in Figure 7–4, it will affect the vowel. The ultrasound images in Figure 7–11—taken from the same sequence—confirm the maintained vowel shape through the /m/. The characteristics of the /ɑ/ (degree of concavity and wave-like shape moving the majority of the volume into the back [posterior] and lowering the tip [apex] to create more resonance space in the front [anterior]; Chapter 5) correspond with the one in the /m/.

Like our various "ah" examples in Chapter 6, it does not look like a "big deal," though looking at the power spectrum (displaying frequency and intensity in vertical lines) of the two different /m/ phonemes, we can clearly see the acoustic outcome (Figure 7–12). The overlay of the gray/red (/m/ sung with CR) and white/green (/m/ sung without CR) lines shows a radical difference in the peaks of $3f_o$ and $4f_o$ (harmonics) in particular due to the change in concavity of the tongue shape. This is to be expected because changes within the mouth (oral) appear around that area. The /m/ with the maintained /ɑ/ shape lowers the peaks, while the /m/ with a convex shape ("hump") increases them. In regard to intensity (determined in part by the height of the peak), you may say that you do want the increased one, and in general, you would be right.

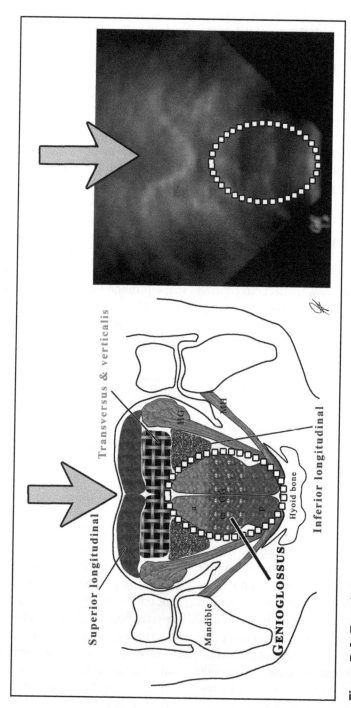

Figure 7–9. Transducer turned 90° for a front (anterior) view of the tongue (*left*), frontal (coronal) cross-sectional graph (*middle*) and ultrasound (*right*). The genioglossus depresses (*white square dotted/yellow oval*), creating the "groove" (*indicated by the arrow*).

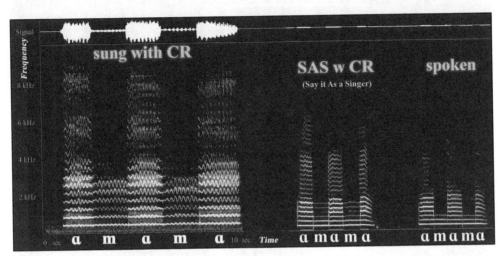

Figure 7–10. Spectrographic comparison of the sequence /amama/ sung, SAS with consonant resonance (CR), and spoken without CR.

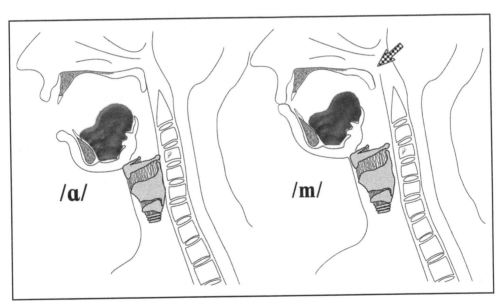

Figure 7–11. Ultrasound images of the tongue shapes taken from the sung sequence /amama/. Note the maintained /ɑ/ shape in the consovowel /m/ and the opening of the uvula (nasopharyngeal port; *arrow*), redirecting the sound through the nose.

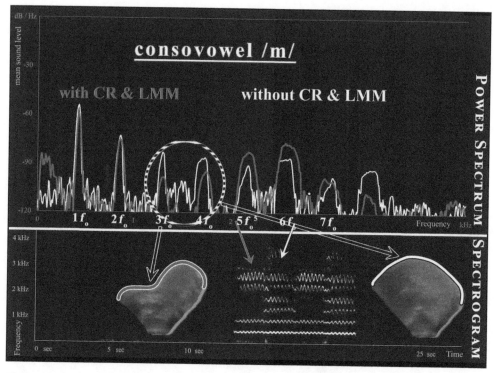

Figure 7–12. Power spectra overlay (*top row*) and corresponding spectrogram (*bottom row*) of the consovowel /m/ sung with consonant resonance (*gray/red*) and without (*white/green*). Note the change of the third and fourth harmonics ($3f_o$, $4f_o$) due to the concomitant tongue shapes.

However, we always need to look at the big picture of acoustic reflection within the entire vocal tract and its articulators (filter).

With that in mind, can you see another part of the overlay showing dissimilarities? Yes, around 5 to $7f_o$ the spectral peaks of the /m/ with CR are now higher. This area, between 2 and 3 kHz (1 kHz = 1000 Hz), constitutes an important component in the overall sound. We call this area the **singer's formant (F_s)** or **singer's formant cluster**, respectively (Sundberg, 1987, 2003), and it is instrumental in the amplification of the voice. Why? On one hand, the sound of an orchestra around this area is fairly weak, whereas the sensitivity of the human ear on the other hand is quite strong. Physiologically, it is created by a lowered larynx, thus extending the laryngeal tube, functioning as

a quasi-autonomous resonator with a resonance frequency in the vicinity of 3 kHz. Of course, this area is of particular interest for singers so they can be heard without amplification even over a very loud orchestra. However, a study that examined the singer's formant and speaker's ring resonance showed that opera singers have more energy concentration not only in their singing but in their speaking voice as well (Lee et al., 2008), hence supporting the SAS concept for actors advocated in this book.

This is why in our /m/ example we have to, in addition to the maintained /ɑ/ tongue shape, keep our larynx in a lowered relaxed position also for maximum acoustic gains. This is accomplished—you guessed it—through the use of the second strategy of the lower mandible maneuver (LMM,

Chapter 3). This drops the back (posterior) of the jaw (mandible) that concomitantly lowers the larynx, creating an extension of the laryngeal tube (Figure 7–13).

Nonpitch (Consonants)

As we have seen over and over during the course of this book, it is never just one element that affects or changes the acoustic outcome. It is the synergy of various settings of our articulators that help us create the maximum CR in every consonant—yes, even those that do not have pitch. Are you skeptical? For some, the concept of CR during the production of pitch consonants (consovowels) may have seemed strange at first though, as we have just seen, more coherent because we are still producing sound due to the vowel component in the consonant. But how does that translate to consonants that do not have any element of vocal fold vibration (nonpitch) and are thus pure noise?

Contrary to the consovowels (pitch consonants) that in the spectrogram show vowel-like harmonics (stacked wave lines; Figure 7–1), the nonpitch consonants are pure noise, as shown in Figure 7–14. What you see are some examples of nonpitch consonants (e.g., /t/ as in "time," /f/ as in "figure," /ç/ as in the German *nicht* [meaning "no/not"], and /tʃ/ as in "church"). The most interesting part is that even though they all appear as noise, they still show their own distinctive signatures. This is because of the way their individually distinct noise components are created, called the **place of articulation** (PoA; we talk more about this second classification of consonants later on).

In the consovowels, we pointed out the critical interaction of the "groove" in the tongue and the relaxed larynx via the LMM for maximum CR production. Continuing on this example, and at the risk of implying an order of importance on it, which I certainly do not intend, this interaction of groove and LMM is even more crucial

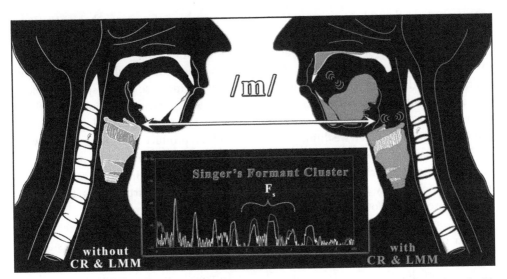

Figure 7–13. Juxtaposition of the sung consovowel /m/ without (*left, white/green*) and with (*right, gray/red*) the low mandible maneuver strategy (Chapter 2). Note the lowered larynx on the right, enabling the clustering of formants within the 3 kHz area, known as the singer's formant cluster.

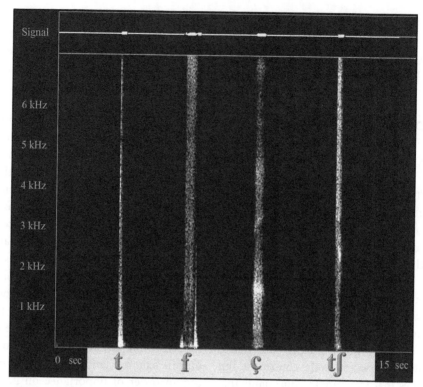

Figure 7–14. Spectrograms of nonpitch consonants. Note that they are all noise yet still show their distinctive signatures.

for resonential balance between vowels and consonants.

We have seen that the tongue root activity is dominated by the genioglossus (GG), which when it depresses, creates this groove and subsequently influences the richness and resonance of the sound (see Figure 7–9 and Chapter 6). Now when we think of nonpitch consonants such as in Figure 7–14, we know that they are formed by obstructing airflow, which is why they are also called obstruent sounds. In other words, we have only the airflow within the vocal tract available to make those consonants audible. How can we do that? You put something in the way of that flow. Try it for yourself: take a breath and exhale at a constant pace through your mouth, like blowing out a magic relighting birthday candle. Now move a finger in and out of that airstream.

Can you hear the noise when your finger moves into/passes through the airstream? This occurs because of the friction that occurs when the air rubs over your finger. When you increase the air speed (by blowing harder), the friction around your finger also increases. This friction between air and object can produce swooshing sounds, what we call *noise*. So, what can we put in the way of the airflow within the vocal tract? Yes, you guessed it, our articulators (tongue, lips, teeth, etc.).

You probably begin to see the challenges that those consonants entail. It is already challenging to get enough resonance in our consovowels (pitch consonants), and that is with the support of sound; in other words, there is no constriction, and all the sound stems from the vibrating (oscillating) vocal folds. In the nonpitch consonants (**obstru-**

ents), we are supposed to achieve the same resonance that rivals our strong vowels solely with airflow. Also, the same applies to what we have said in the consovowels discussion and in Chapter 1 for the nonpitch consonants: they carry much (if not most) of the burden of dramatic interpretation in singing/acting. They are vital for musical and articulatory reasons that include but are not limited to accentuating/emphasizing the meaning of a word, rhythm, volume, and/ or personal interpretation. Remember our example from Chapter 1? Take, for example, the word *fiammate* ("inflame" in English) at the end of the phrase, where the word initial /f/ was significantly lengthened. Or how about some Hamlet? In Act 2, Scene 2, Polonius reads the letter with the first line: "Doubt thou the stars are fire, [. . .]" ("You

may wonder if the stars are fire"). I am sure the /f/ in "fire" could benefit from some lengthening as well, not to mention what we could and have to do, for intelligibility, with the preceding consonants in that line.

Because they do not have a pitch, the biggest challenge of nonpitch consonants is that their excitation in the vocal tract occurs much higher than at the glottis (space between vocal folds; see Figure 7–2). Thus, a *shorter* vocal tract is excited. More precisely, the lower-frequency resonance is canceled by antiresonances of the back cavity of the vocal tract; therefore, higher resonances appear in the speech spectra. You can imagine that this is not ideal for projection in singing/acting.

Have a look at Figure 7–15. On the left, you can see the spectrogram of /ʃɑ/ ("sh" as

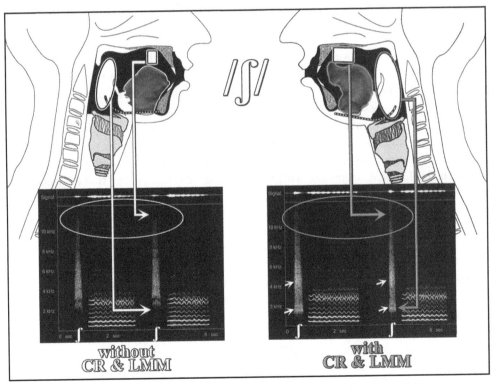

Figure 7–15. Juxtaposition of tongue shape and spectrogram of the consonant /ʃ/ (as in shine). In the spectrogram, note the differences in higher frequencies (*oval*), formants (*arrows*), and the cleaner consonant-to-vowel transition with consonant resonance and low mandible maneuver (*right*).

in "shine" and /ɑ/ as in "law") sung without CR and LMM as well as the corresponding tongue position of the consonant /ʃ/. On the right, we have the same but now with the desired CR and applied LMM. As we have already seen in Chapters 4 and 6, in the two tongue shapes, the hump on the left indicates that there is no groove in the front of the tongue, whereas the dimple on the right implies that a groove is present. And, like in Figure 7–12, follow the gray/red line in the right suggesting the applied LMM (jaw is dropped in the back; posterior mandible drop) and the one on the left, without LMM.

Until now, we have always had a pitch component, but let us put all the previously introduced puzzle pieces (LMM, 2D/3D tongue shapes, source filter theory, etc.) together and look at their effects on the resonance of consonants without pitch (noise) (see Figure 7–15). Starting with the "hump versus groove," you can see that if there is a hump (no groove, left), the line of the /ʃ/ in the spectrogram does not show the higher frequencies that we can see on the right image, where the tongue concavity indicates a groove. Further on, the production of the consonants without LMM also shows fewer lower frequencies versus the one with the LMM. Continuing with the analyses, most of the time formants are dismissed within consonants because they are not very prominent and are extremely scattered, making them hard to analyze. However, the image on the right with the applied CR and LMM shows the contrary (arrows). And last but certainly not least, we can see that the beginning of the vowel (/ɑ/) in the left is not as exact, showing some inconsistency before turning into steady wave lines. All of these differences are not only clearly audible but also visible in numbers in the more detailed spectrogram of Voce Vista (Figure 7–16).

Why is it critical to have *both* CR and LMM, and what is the acoustic process behind it? The LMM prevents the lower frequencies from being cancelled out by antiresonances of the back cavity of the vocal tract. The "groove" on the other hand creates a narrow passage that functions as a Venturi tube (**Venturi effect**) (i.e., accelerating the airflow, which breaks against the teeth to produce the high-frequency turbulence associated with the fricative /ʃ/), but that is not all. Larger halls or churches with long reverberation are intolerable at high pitches, and in acoustically challenged spaces we need every bit of intensity, resonance, and frequency spectrum to ensure the presence of our voice and consonants in particular.

Et voilà! Another secret is revealed. Keeping the two-chamber hallway metaphor introduced in Chapter 5, even though we have no pitch, we need to make sure that the airstream does get ample resonance space in those chambers. Although part of the tongue moving into the front (anterior) chamber (like in our /ʃ/ example), we ought to keep in mind the hydrostatic and 3D characteristics of the tongue (like having a little groove in the front part of tongue) to ensure that all physical and physioacoustic forces behind that airstream can be set and utilized in the most effective, desired manner.

In summary, it can be said that with applied CR and LMM,

- there are more higher *and* lower frequencies in the nonpitch consonant,
- there are more prominent and less scattered formants,
- there is a cleaner transition from the consonant to the vowel, and
- an increase in amplitude can be measured.

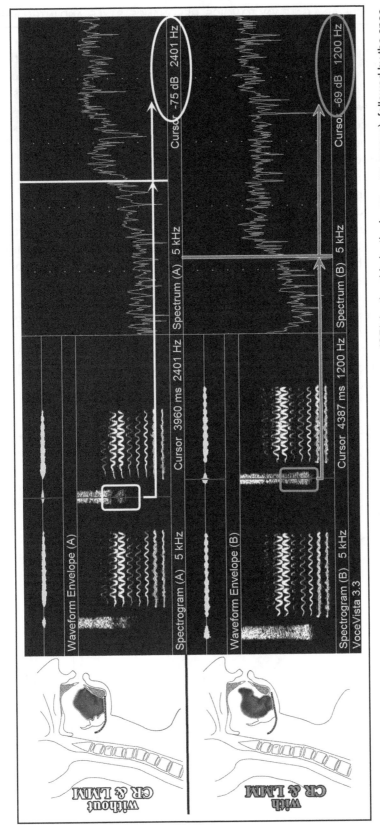

Figure 7–16. *Top left to right:* Ultrasound of the fricative /ʃ/ without consonant resonance (CR) (noticeable by the hump = no groove), followed by the spectrogram (Voce Vista). *Bottom left to right:* Ultrasound of the fricative /ʃ/ with CR (noticeable by the dimple = groove) and spectrograph measurements.

Place of Articulation

In Chapter 5, we briefly talked about the articulation of consonants. In general, and as we just saw in the CR, they involve some degree of obstruction in the form of closure or near-closure of the vocal tract. Let us slowly say the consonants /k/ (complement), /p/ (pastry), and /g/ (gorgeous). All three involve a momentarily complete blockage of the airway with either the tongue or the lips. Because of that momentary closure, the airway is considered closed, even if just for a split second.

Now, say these consonants from another phonemic class, /s/ (sun), /ʃ/ (show), and /f/ (fabulous); notice that even though there is no complete blockage of airflow, your articulators (teeth and/or lips) allow only a min-

iscule gap through which air can flow. This tiny aperture causes the airflow to become turbulent and create noise. This almost-stoppage is also considered a closed vocal tract because the action can be sustained (try it out: it is easy to sustain a /ʃ/ for 5 sec or more).

This brings us to the **place of articulation (PoA).** The **articulation** is a formation of articulators necessary within the vocal tract for clear and distinct sounds. The **place** is to which these articulators are corresponding with, from the front of the vocal tract to the back (Figure 7–17). The more mobile parts of the vocal tract, such as lips and tongue, are **active PoAs,** contrary to the **passive PoA,** which is more stationary and composed from parts anywhere from the upper teeth, gums, or roof of the mouth to the back of the throat.

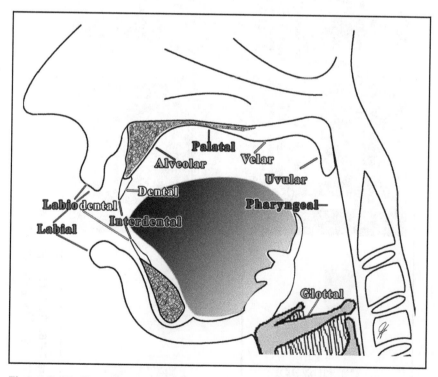

Figure 7–17. The relationships between the articulators and their corresponding places of articulation.

However, as singers/actors and through the lens of maximum resonance in all phonemes, we ought to reconsider and modify some standardized PoA. Although we are focusing on the place to which the articulators are corresponding, sometimes it is hard to know what part within an articulator is chosen to correspond to the PoA.

For example, the phoneme /ʒ/ (voiced "sh" as in beige) can sometimes be found classified as palatal, postalveolar, palatoalveolar, and so forth. It is a question on how specific one wants to be in regard to the tongue's actual or near contact to the palate. However, in our example, the edges of the tongue body (dorsum of the tongue) touch a relatively large area from the middle to the back of the upper teeth, and the tip is only approximate to the alveolar ridge.

We should also consider the individual tongue shapes a person can have. Not everyone has the same tongue, which can range from a short to a long tongue or even a tongue-tie (ankyloglossia; can vary in degree of severity from mild to complete ankyloglossia, whereby the tongue is tethered to the floor of the mouth). Any of them can change the PoA in order to ensure the accuracy of the phoneme.

Either way, you will soon see the regions are not strictly separated and may overlap or change for some consonants depending on the prerequisites of both the demands of resonance creation and individual tongue shapes.

Labials: Sounds are produced by one or both lips

Let us start from the front of our vocal tract: the lips. Anything that relates or is adjacent to the lips is called *labial*. The /l/ correlates to the word **lips** (Latin word for lips is *labium*). Sounds that are produced by one or both lips (/p/, /b/, /f/, /v/, /m/, and /ʷ/ [Figure 7–18]) resulting in a partial or complete closure are **labial.** If both the lower and upper lips are combined, we get **bilabial** sounds, such as /b/ (boat), /p/ (pin), /ʷ/ (what), /m/ (mother), and so forth. Raising the lower lip to contact the upper teeth

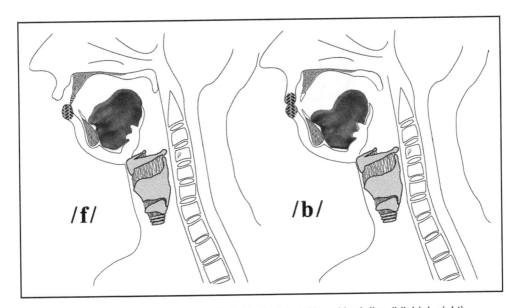

Figure 7–18. Lower lip and upper teeth (labiodental, *left*) and both lips (bilabial, *right*).

produces the **labiodentals**, such as /f/ (funny) and /v/ (voice).

Dentals, Interdentals, or Linguadentals: Tongue contacts the teeth

Dental, interdental, or linguadental sounds arise when the tongue contacts the teeth. A **dental** consonant is considered to be articulated with the tongue against the upper teeth, such as /t/, /d/, /n/, and /l/ in some languages. Dentals are usually distinguished from sounds in which contact is made with the tongue and the gum ridge, as in English (see alveolar) because of the acoustic similarity of the sounds. There are dentals that can be found in some dialect of American English (Edwards, 2003). However, only two sounds are typically considered as dental across the dialects of American English—the interdentals, /θ/ (with) and /ð/ (that) (Figure 7–19).

Alveolar: Tongue contacts the area behind the upper teeth

Alveolar consonants, which are called that because they contain the sockets (the alveoli) of the upper teeth, are articulated when the tongue typically contacts the area behind the upper teeth (alveolar ridge). Particular in American English, we find a lot of consonants with their PoA (placeof articulation) in this area, for example, /t/, /d/, /s/, /z/, /n/, /l/ (Figure 7–20). Try them out and feel where the tip of the tongue (apex) establishes contact. Are you touching some teeth as well? It is a very narrow margin between teeth and alveolar, and depending on the opening of the mouth, or jaw (mandible), respectively, as well as the shape and length of your tongue tip, the PoA may move more toward the teeth or the alveolar ridge (start of the hard palate) (see Figure 7–20). Later, we explore in more detail the possible

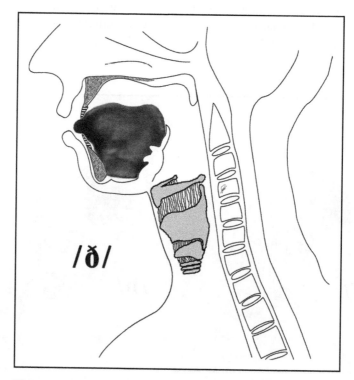

Figure 7–19. Tongue tip between both teeth (dental).

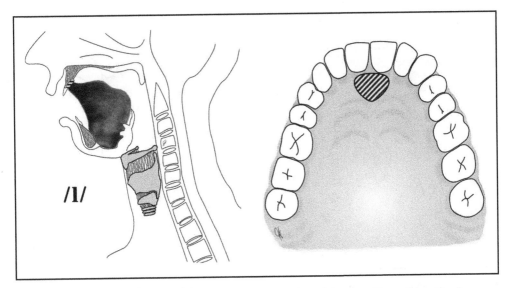

Figure 7–20. Tip of the tongue touches upper front palate (alveolar ridge, *striped/red*).

options within every consonant, such as the /t/. Other consonants, such as /r/, /ʃ/, and /ʒ/, may not have complete closure but are in close proximity with the tip of the tongue (apex) toward the alveolar ridge.

Palatal: Tongue contacts part of the hard palate, or roof of the mouth.

Moving farther back, we are progressing into the larger area of the hard palate or roof of the mouth. Because it is relatively large, one may subdivide it into **alveopalatals, prepalatals, palatals,** and **postpalatals.** As we see later (see Manner of Articulation), some consonant sounds are stops (airflow is stopped completely and then released) or a combination of an initial stop and partial blockage, such as affricates. If you take the word *judge* (/d̠ʒʌd̠ʒ/) and very slowly SAS it (meaning say it with resonance), you will find (a) an initial block of airflow in the /d/ (an alveolar consonant, starting with the tip of the tongue [apex] behind the top teeth while sealing with the edge of the tongue along the upper teeth the oral cavity) and (b) a release of the built-up pressure turn-

ing into a turbulent, hence noisy airflow through the teeth. Thus, phonetically the /dʒ/ would be considered an alveopalatal consonant (d = alveolar, ʒ = palatal). Other palatals are /ʃ/, /ʒ/, /tʃ/, /dʒ/, /ʲ/, and some productions of /r/.

Of course, in German, as well as in other languages, we have pure palatal consonants, for example, /ç/ (El<u>ch</u>, German for "elk/moose"). In Figure 7–21 (left), you can see the tongue moving up vertically. An important part to note here is that it is not the actual contact of the tongue to the palate. We need to remind ourselves of the 3D nature of the tongue that unfortunately is not possible to show within this image. The rounding on top can be deceiving, indicating a contact of the middle of the tongue with the palate, whereas in fact only the edges are touching the palate. In other words, we have a region along the outer side of the palate (Figure 7–21, right) as our PoA and a midline groove along the tongue. This phoneme is not to be confused with the guttural /χ/, as we discuss in the next paragraph.

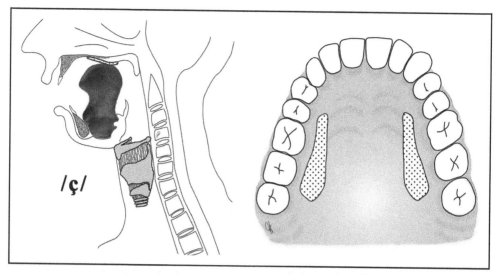

Figure 7–21. Dots/ Green indicating contact of the tongue edges on upper palatal region in the side view (*left*) and the upper palate (*right*).

Velar: Tongue contacts the soft palate (velum)

Sliding along the palate with the tip of the tongue (apex), we can feel a bit of a bump farther back, which marks the transition from hard to soft palate, and then dips into the soft tissue of the velum. The sounds made with tongue contact on or about the soft palate (**velum**) are /k/, /g/, and /ŋ/. However, other sounds whose primary PoA is near the back of the oral cavity are also called **guttural** sounds. The term was primarily used for pharyngeal consonants, hence the word *guttural* (from the Latin *guttur*, meaning "throat"). Contrasting to the palatal sound /ç/ we discussed in the previous paragraph, the PoA of the guttural /χ/ (A<u>ch</u>!, German for "alas") phoneme is the soft palate, uvula and can be found in languages such as German, Russian, African, and Dutch. The friction created between the back of the tongue and uvular may be perceived as a harsh, heavy, and/or throaty sound, particularly for those whose language does not have such sounds.

In German, there is a particular confusion in both when to use the palate /ç/ or the guttural /χ/ and how to make those sounds. As you can see in Figure 7–22, the PoA is more in the back of the soft palate region. Compared to Figure 7–21, the differences are apparent in the shape of the tongue as well as the PoA. Unfortunately, there has been some controversy concerning when to use one or the other. In Part II of this book where I provide instructions for each individual consonant, I add a brief discussion about some of the current problems in German pronunciation and hopefully help clarify the discrepancies surrounding some consonants.

Glottal: Does not have an actual PoA but uses partial closure or close approximation of the vocal folds for some friction or turbulence. The space between the vocal folds is called the *glottis*, and the phoneme produced by narrowing that space is /h/. However, in singing and acting, we need to exaggerate. In the case of the /h/, this exag-

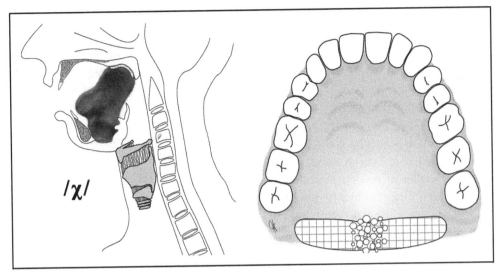

Figure 7–22. Tiles/Pink indicating contact of the tongue edges on upper palatal region in the side view (*left*) and the upper palate (*right*).

geration could be both exhausting and possibly tensing up the larynx. Under that lens, I am suggesting a palatal addition in the production of the /h/ sound by some narrowing of the oral cavity with the tongue, creating extra turbulence (more detail on that in Part II).

Manner of Articulation

So far, we have talked about two of the three criteria to describe consonant sounds: (a) the voicing (pitch versus nonpitch) and (b) the PoA. Last, but not least, we have to talk about the **manner of articulation (MoA)**, which refers to *how* the airflow is constricted. As mentioned earlier, moving the PoA may be necessary not only to accommodate the shape of an individual tongue or a more open and relaxed jaw position but also to change the resonance of the consonant (CR). With the MoA, the positioned articulators are also able to con-

trol the flow of the air or both air and sound through the vocal tract. This can range from a complete stop to only a partial blockage of airflow. So, what are the most common manners of articulation to describe consonants?

Stops/Plosives

As the word implies, these sounds are made with a complete blockage of airflow followed by a release of that air. Of course, the release itself can also range from an audible burst of air to one that is barely noticeable. How? Take for instance the phoneme /p/ as in plosive. Say it twice: for the first time, keep your lips sealed, build up the pressure behind it (like in a cartoon, where the head swells up and turns red before it explodes) and then release it. Did you hear the extreme burst of air after the release? Now, do the same thing but without the exaggeration of the pressure buildup. Did you notice how minor the burst is compared to the first time? Because of the burst of air, they are also referred to as **plosives.** Other examples are /b/, /t/, /d/, /k/, and /g/ (Figure 7–23).

Fricatives

Contrary to the stops/plosives, fricative sounds are created by a partial blockage of airflow where the tongue approaches but does not make contact with a PoA. Like we discussed earlier in this chapter, this creates a bottleneck of airflow by narrowing the space between the articulator and PoA, causing, as the word implies, a friction-like sound such as /ʃ/, /ʒ/, /f/, /v/, /θ/, and /ð/ (Figure 7–24).

Affricates

These sounds are composed of two different manners in the sequence of stop and fricative. In other words, it starts with a stop and is released as fricative in rapid succession. For instance, the phoneme /tʃ/ (chair) starts with the stop /t/ (tag) and is immediately released into the fricative /ʃ/ (shine) (Figure 7–25).

Nasals: The **nasal** sounds are produced when the air is redirected through the nose by lowering the velum. How do you know that the velum is open instead of closed? Hold the phoneme /m/ (moon) and then close your nose with your fingers. Did the sound stop? That is because the air is only going through the nasal cavity while the rest is sealed off by the lips. Other nasals are /n/ and /ŋ/ (Figure 7–26).

Liquids: This is a generic term for consonants where the air, or in this case sound, can pass on one or both sides of the tongue,

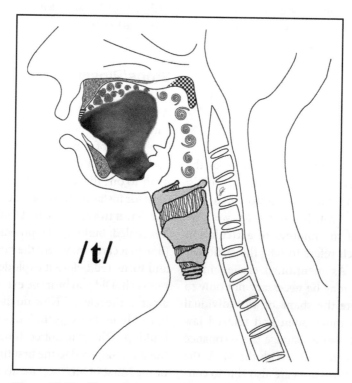

/t/

Figure 7–23. Air particles blocked before being released.

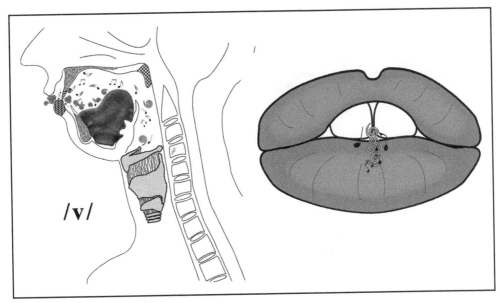

Figure 7–24. Sound and air particles escape only through a narrow-centered opening between the upper teeth and lower lip.

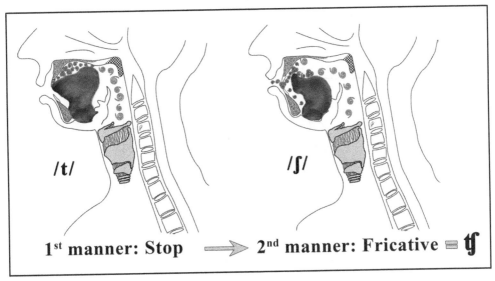

Figure 7–25. Two successive manners creating the phoneme /tʃ/ (catch).

such as the American English /l/ (land) and /ɹ/ (red) sounds (Figure 2–27).

Glides: As we discussed in Chapter 6, **glides** are like "reversed" diphthongs in which the secondary (shorter of the two) transitory vowel is performed first. These consonants (Figure 7–28) do not have any constriction, which is also why they are called semivowels, such as /ʷ/ (what) and /ʲ/ (yes).

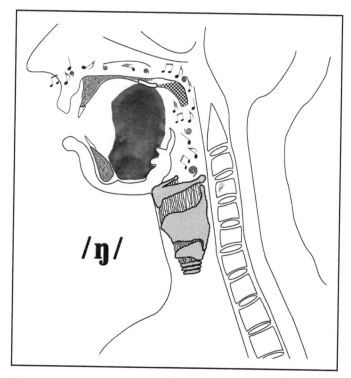

Figure 7–26. Air particles with sound are moving through the nasal cavity.

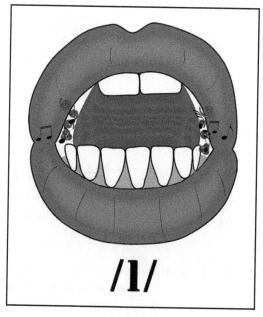

Figure 7–27. Air particles with sound passing on both sides (front view [coronal]).

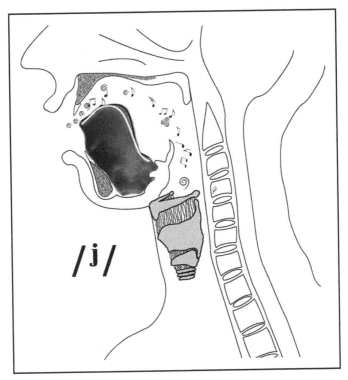

Figure 7–28. No constriction during the indicated glide (*black/ red and white/green lines*).

Taps: As the word implies, the tap results when an active articulator, such as the tongue, throws itself (like a rapid flick) against a passive articulator, such as the upper teeth or the upper gum ridge (alveolar ridge). In American English, the tap or flap is commonly used for some productions of the middle /t/ as in le**tt**er or the /d/ as in la**dd**er. In other words, instead of making a full stop for the /t/ in letter (/lɛtɚ/), in North America we only flick the tongue tip against the upper gum ridge (/lɛɾɚ/).

Now, do you need to take a breath after all these details? I am very aware that it can be quite overwhelming at first looking at phonemes and particularly consonants in such a meticulous manner. However, every one of these little details helps amateurs and professionals improve their personal or professional work, making the execution much easier and subsequently enabling everyone to use the entire potential of their voice. I believe that it is fascinating, how we are able to execute all of these seemingly minor details without even thinking about them (at least in regular speech).

I encourage you to dive into those details. Consonants are the spine of the word. They are crucial for intelligibility and give rhythm and emotional content. Now, what we need to do is put into action all the theoretical key ingredients that we have been talking about (Figure 7–29):

- LMM,
- tongue movement, and
- voicing/PoA/MoA.

We then have the secret to exploiting the full range of every single phoneme, in every

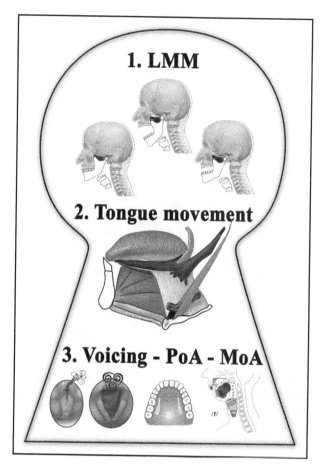

Figure 7–29. Theoretical key ingredients.

word of every sentence, whether for speech or singing, with or without a microphone. Let us start the intriguing and very rewarding step-by-step process of how to modify them, so you are equipped with the tools to ensure intelligibility, while conveying the message with your interpretation and emotions.

References

Edwards, H. T. (2003). *Applied phonetics: The sounds of American English* (3rd ed.). Clifton Park, NY: Thomson.

Fant, G. (1960). *Acoustic theory of speech production*. The Hague, Netherlands: Mouton.

Fujimura, O. (1962). Analysis of nasal consonants. *Journal of the Acoustical Society of America, 34,* 1865–1875.

Henderson, C., & Palmer C. (1940). *How to sing for money.* New York, NY: Harcourt, Brace.

Ladefoged, P., Maddieson, I., (1996) *The sounds of the world's languages.* Malden, MA: Blackwell Publisher.

Lee, S-H., Kwon, H-J., Choi, H-J., Lee, N-H., Lee, S-J., & Jin, S-M. (2008). The singer's formant and speaker's ring resonance: A long-term average spectrum analysis. *Clinical and Experimental Otorhinolaryngology, 1*(2), 92–96.

Miller, D. G. (2008). *Resonance in singing. Voice building through acoustic feedback.* Princeton, NJ: Inside View Press.

Nair, G. (1999). *Voice, tradition and technology.* San Diego, CA: Singular Publishing.

Nair, G. (2007). *The craft of singing.* San Diego, CA: Plural Publishing.

Peterson, G. E., & Barney, H. L. (1952). Control methods used in a study of the vowels. *Journal of the Acoustical Society of America, 24*(2), 175.

Recasens, D. (1983). Place cues for nasal consonants with special reference to Catalan. *Journal of the Acoustical Society of America, 73*(4), 1346–1353.

Sataloff, R. T. (2005). *Professional voice: The science and art of clinical care* (3rd ed.). San Diego, CA: Plural Publishing.

Sundberg, J. (1987). *The science of the singing voice.* Dekalb, IL: Northern Illinois University Press.

Sundberg, J. (2003). Research on the singing voice in retrospect. *TMH-Quarterly Progress and Status Report, 45,* 11–22.

Titze, I. (2000). *Principles of voice production* (2nd ed.). Iowa City, IA: National Center for Voice and Speech.

Titze, I., Baken, R. J., Bozeman, K. W., Granqvist, S., Henrich, N., Herbst, C. T., . . . Wolfe, J. (2015). Toward a consensus on symbolic notation of harmonics, resonances, and formants in vocalization. *Journal of the Acoustical Society of America, 137*(5), 3005–3007.

Titze, I., & Verdolini-Abbott, K. (2012). *Vocology: The science and practice of voice habilitation.* Salt Lake City, UT: National Center for Voice and Speech.

PART II

Applied Knowledge

Introduction

In the first part of this book, we built our knowledge on a more theoretical basis. Now, we see how we can actually apply this knowledge to the most common consonants that one can find in English, Italian, German, and/or French.

Before we get started, a few notes are in order: This book is for singers, actors, speakers, and anyone interested in achieving greater projection, intelligibility, and variability, particularly through consonant resonance, ensuring equal resonance to both vowels and consonants.

Now, some actors and actresses may already know Arthur Lessac's book *The Use and Training of the Human Voice* (1994) and ask what the difference between his and this book may be. First, Lessac is one of the few artists who early on started to pay more attention to the consonants. Drawn from his personal experiences as a teacher and performer, his approach to improve the consonants is based on what he calls *The Consonant Orchestra,* connecting each consonant to the action of a specific musical instrument and its accompanied sensation.

However, with the knowledge and images from the ultrasound, we are able to tap even deeper into the world of consonants, giving precise instructions—based on physiology—on how to maneuver every articulator, particularly the tongue. So, for those who are already familiar with Lessac's approach, this book will be a wonderful toolbox for going deeper into the physiology, achieving maximum consonant resonance, and subsequently reaching a broader acoustic spectrum for a variety of creative expressions. Others who start with this book may want to augment their knowledge with Lessac's approach, as well as sentences, poems, and other explorative selections particularly tailored to acting.

As for the instructions, please keep in mind that we are all individuals, hence no tongue is the same. This is why the following instructions on the shape of the tongue and the place of articulation (PoA) have to be seen as suggestions and approximations. For instance, for someone with a very short tongue, ensuring maximum consonant resonance (CR) for the phoneme /l/ may mean that their ideal PoA of the tongue tip may be a bit more on the backside of the gum ridge (alveolar) or the beginning of the hard palate than at the front. Some of those encounters are discussed in the Common Challenges section along with some of the difficulties in executing the step-by-step instructions so that individual modifications can be made.

Also, occasionally, we refer to a spectrogram. It is a wonderful tool for voice analysis in research, vocal training, and therapy. The instructions provided in this book are based on pedagogical methods that have been proven helpful in my personal studio and, of course, are tailored specifically to consonants. However, if you want to learn more about the general use of a sound spectrograph and how it can be used in the service of one's own pedagogical approach in the voice, I refer you to Garyth Nair's book *Voice Tradition and Technology* (1999). Also, Scott McCoy's *Your Voice: An Inside View* (2012), Kenneth Bozeman's *Practical Vocal Acoustic* (2013), and Donald Miller's *Resonance in Singing* (2008) are other texts that embrace the objective understanding of voice and singing and provide information on how to apply it through the real-time feedback of spectrography.

Finally, there are some "golden rules," if you will, that have experientially proven to be of tremendous help in making the production of consonants, or any phoneme for that matter, easier and freeing the voice. So, should you find yourself becoming stiff and tight, try to think of them as a checklist and see if they make the execution of the consonants easier.

■ **Separate articulation from phonation/ sound.** The principle of the source-filter theory (see Chapter 5): the vocal folds are creating the sound (source is the fundamental frequency), which is the same no matter what phoneme you are producing. The articulators (tongue, lips, jaw, teeth, and various combinations of them) are responsible for the creation of the phoneme (filter). Thus, no additional muscular action is required, particularly from the larynx, if either a change of timbre and/or phoneme (e.g., dark-bright, /e/-/ɑ/) or the creation of noise (such as the hissing of the consonant /s/) is desired.

■ **Let physics work for you.** Think of what the characteristics (manner of articulation) of the consonants are: sound, noise, or both. Then, think through the physiology:

■ Which one of the articulators is involved?

■ How are they collaborating with each other? (Are they creating a place of articulation together? Are they in close proximity and/or narrowing the vocal tract and some point?) and

■ Once everything is set, direct the momentum of the consonant's "explosion" or "constriction" backward instead of pushing it farther outward. You are feeling a backpressure that expands all soft membranes (tongue, soft palate, palatoglossus, etc.), like blowing up a balloon (Figure II–1).

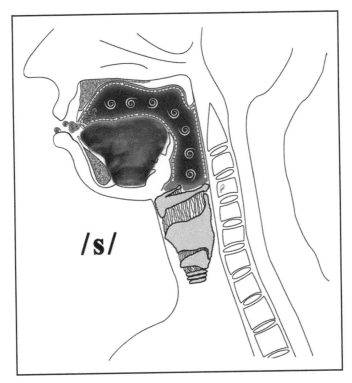

/s/

Figure II–1. Air pressure (*circles/blue*) expands soft membranes and strokes along various surfaces in the mouth (oro-) and throat (pharyngeal) cavity (*arrows/red*).

▪ **Keep moving, step by step.** Focusing on particular actions, such as moving the back of the tongue up to the uvula while keeping the tip of the tongue down and a little retracted, is quite complex. The tongue is able to extend and retract at the same time because extrinsic and intrinsic muscles together provide independent parameters that give the tongue incredible freedom to move and form itself in a three-dimensional shape. At first, this can be quite an overwhelming task, leading to a complete blockage not only in the tongue but also the jaw, larynx, neck, and so forth, by contracting the muscles.

In the following chapters, step-by-step instructions to each consonant are presented to help you focus on one task at a time. However, to avoid a complete freeze by the end of the instructions, you may want to push the reset button at any time along the instructions by (a) shaking off any tension with the entire body, (b) circling with the jaw (Figure II–2, left), and (c) moving the tongue around the mouth and biting on it (like a massage). Also, wiggling the head sideways (left and right) with small motions (like drawing a line with your nose only 1/16-inch-long will help to free up the laryngeal and suboccipital muscles in particular (Figure II–2, right).

▪ **Trigger Points.** *Note:* The following instructions are not only useful to release tension while singing/speaking but are highly advisable to use as a warm-up regimen before singing/speaking.

Trigger points can be viewed in a similar manner to the focused movement of muscles. Only now we are stimulating or massaging specific points with our fingers from the outside, instead of moving them within their skeletal function from the inside (cir-

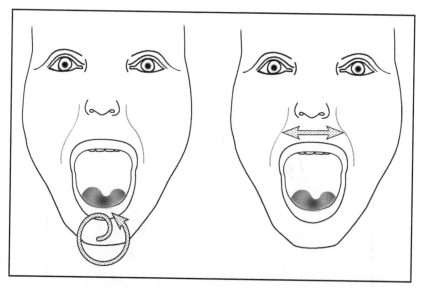

Figure II–2. Rotate jaw clockwise and counterclockwise (*left*) and wiggle left and right with your head (*right*) as relaxation while doing the exercise and/or between each exercise.

cling the jaw). How should you massage? In general, the intensity should be strong enough to satisfy but easy to bear. Thus, we want the "good pain." Now, have a look at Figure II–3 and start in the indicated numeral order:

1. With your index and middle fingers (or middle and ring) at the bottom edge of the jaw, find the knot that hurts. With small circles, start to put on pressure and slowly increase the diameter. See if you notice a release along the jaw, even neck, on the outside and almost through the entire vocal tract in the inside (like the bottom of the tongue).

2. Find the hinge in front of each ear (temporomandibular joint [TMJ]) and move above the bone. This is where the temporalis muscle starts and then spreads out like a fan. Take three to four fingers, start to massage at the bottom area with small circles, and finish every cycle by moving up along the entire muscle. Do you notice any release around the muscle, within the TMJ and entire jaw?

3. Under the hinge in front of each ear you can find a notch in the cheekbone.

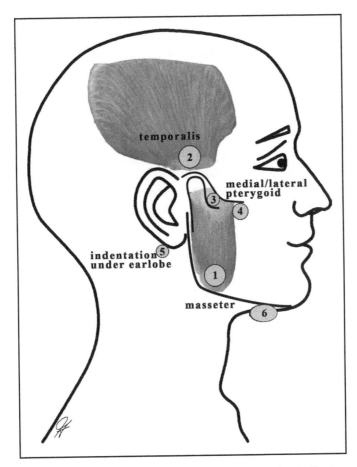

Figure II–3. Various trigger points to release tension in the jaw and subsequently the larynx, tongue, neck, and so on.

With your fingertip or thumb, press firmly inward and upward, simulating circle motions. Do you feel the sweet ache of release? If you want to really dig deep and get a good release, the best way to massage is to put your thumb inside your mouth and knead the muscle between your thumb and fingers.

4. From the previous position, move along the cheekbone and find the next point and continue with either constant pressure or small, kneading circles.

5. This is a functional point to relieve jaw tension and is located in the indentation under the earlobe. Using your middle fingers, start to apply light pressure to stimulate the point. Because this point can often be tender, be gentle with the pressure and do not forget to breathe when doing it as a warm-up. It is a great point to tone fascial muscles, treat lockjaw, relieve jaw pain, and so on.

6. Take all the fingers you have and start kneading the triangle (mylo-, genio-hyoid; see Chapter 2) under your jaw. Notice any release, particularly in the tongue. Then, with both thumbs side by side, slide them from the bottom part of the chin straight toward the larynx. After a few repetitions, continue by sliding more toward the side along the jawbone, almost back to your ears.

In general, anything we do—may it be a touch, massage, movement, or the like—should always have some sort of effect. For instance, when you massage, try to be sensitive to changes, such as relief, tickle, or even "good" pain right at the spot, or radiated throughout the area, the entire skull, maybe even the upper body (shoulders, etc.). No matter what the outcome, it is about taking notice to build awarness of the status quo, which in turn allows us to learn to either improve or, if necessary, change it to make the process easier.

For anyone interested in the science of trigger points as well as trigger point therapy for the entire body, I highly recommend Davies and Davies's *The Trigger Point Therapy Workbook* (2013) and Uppgaard's *Taking Control of TMJ* (1999).

The images in Figures II–4 to II–7 provide a visual reference to facilitate a clear understanding of the various instructions in the chapters to follow.

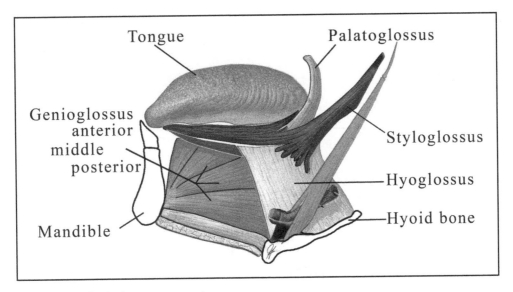

Figure II–4. Extrinsic tongue muscles.

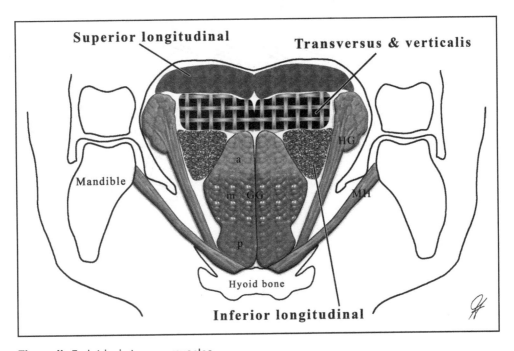

Figure II–5. Intrinsic tongue muscles.

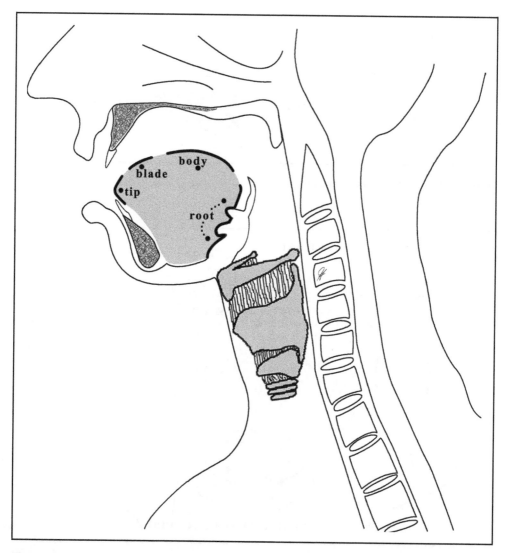

Figure II–6. Tongue parts.

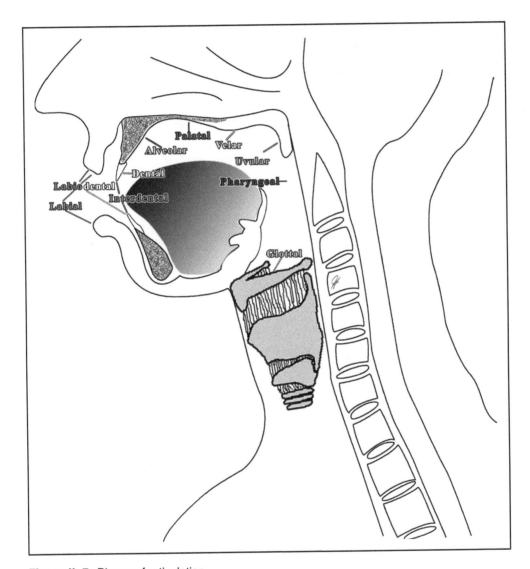

Figure II–7. Places of articulation.

References

Bozeman, K. W. (2013). *Practical vocal acoustics.* Vox Musicae: The Voice, Vocal Pedagogy, and Song. Series No. 9.

Davies, C., & Davies, A. (2013). *The trigger point therapy workbook. Your self-treatment guide for pain relief* (3rd ed.). Oakland, CA: New Harbinger Publications.

Edwards, H. T. (2003). *Applied phonetics: The sounds of American English* (3rd ed.). Clifton Park, NY: Thomson.

Lessac, A. (1994). *The use and training of the human voice. A bio-dynamic approach to vocal life* (3rd ed.). New York, NY: McGraw Hill Higher Education.

McCoy, S. (2012). *Your voice: An inside view* (2nd ed.). Gahanna, OH: Inside View Press.

Miller, D. G. (2008). *Resonance in singing. Voice building through acoustic feedback.* Princeton, NJ: Inside View Press.

Nair, G. (1999). *Voice, tradition and technology.* San Diego, CA: Singular Publishing

Uppgaard, R. O. (1999). *Taking control of TMJ. Your total wellness program for recovering from temporomandibular joint pain, whiplash, fibromyalgia, and related disorders.* Oakland, CA: New Harbinger Publications.

8 Nasal and Continuant Consonants— /m/ /n/ /ŋ/ /ɲ/ /l/

General Considerations

As the word implies, the nasal consonants are produced by a complete closure at some place along the length of the mouth (oral) region of the vocal tract (from the lips in the front to the velum in the back). However, unlike in stop consonants, such as /p/, /t/, and so forth (see Chapter 7), we do not feel a pressure increase behind the closure because the uvula (velopharyngeal port) is open. Let us try it out and feel the difference.

Before we start though, a note of caution is in order: The pressure difference between the middle ear and the outside, if not released, can result in a burst eardrum. Therefore, the following exercise should be done very carefully and not by any means fast and/or pushed. Close your mouth and keep breathing through your nose. Then exhale in slow motion and gently pinch your nose closed. Release immediately. Could you feel how the pressure inside increases when you close your nose? Of course, with consonants, the feeling is less extreme, but it is all about increasing the awareness for any pressure change.

In Chapter 6 we saw that some consonants have more vowel-like qualities compared to others. This is certainly the case in our nasals. Unlike the fricatives (e.g., /f/

= flower) that result from a degree of vocal tract turbulence (noise), the nasals /m/ /n/ /ŋ/ /ɲ/ depend more on pitch (voicing) and resonance. We do not pay much attention to it when we speak because the voicing of the nasals is so short that they are easily dismissed. Just quickly say the word "mammoth" (/mæməθ/) and then repeat it in slow motion, giving each phoneme at least 2 sec. Did you want to stop the phonation on the /m/ just right after the first onset of sound?

This is not surprising because when we speak, we do not sustain the voiced consonant. But with the uninterrupted outward airflow, the vocal folds start to vibrate (oscillation), which in turn creates a sound (Chapter 7); this means that they have pitch that we can sustain. By slowing down the phonation, we notice the voicing in our speech. Thus, nasals behave more like vowels and should be treated as such in both speaking and singing. Of course, in singing it means that we are able to continue singing the melody line by sustaining the pitch the nasal is assigned to. Furthermore, this is the reason we need to make sure to modify them in the same manner as we do with the vowels, particularly when ascending into the *passaggi* (transitions; Chapter 7). Which vowel should you use, you may ask? In general, depending on the distribution of the nasals in the word—initial, middle, final—the preceding or following vowel of the nasal is the one to consider for both resonance creation and/or modification.

Thinking of nasals as vowels will also help to create maximum consonant resonance (CR) and subsequently assure their projection as well as the continuation of the resonance of vowels. The overall amplitude of nasals is usually less than that of adjacent vowels. As a result, they almost seem to disappear. Because airflow of nasals is going through the nasal cavity and out the nostrils, the oral cavity becomes more like a side chamber. In Chapter 7, we discussed that we need to work with both pharyngeal and oral cavities so that antiresonances are not cancelling out higher or lower frequencies. Remember the two-hallway metaphor in Chapter 5? The tongue with its various shapes creates two "rooms" with the con-

necting "hallway" (the narrowest space between tongue surface and roof of the mouth). The relative shape and size of the two "rooms" are the acoustic reasons that each of these phonemes sound the way they do. In the case of the nasal /m/ (Figure 8–1), the oral cavity is the side chamber that can either amplify the resonance by being as open as possible (more lowered position of the tongue apex and body through the groove in front; right image) or cancel it out by antiresonances with the cavity blocked by a more upward, higher position of the tongue and larynx (dimple in the front of the tongue; left image) (see also Chapters 6 and 7).

But I am getting ahead of myself. Let us first start with the articulatory considerations of the nasal /m/ (see Figure 8–1).

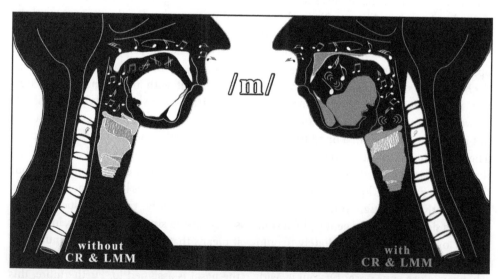

Figure 8–1. Juxtaposition of the nasal /m/ with and without consonant resonance (CR). The sound travels through the nose and also reflects in the oral and pharyngeal cavities; if blocked by a more upward, higher position of the tongue and larynx (dimple in the front of the tongue (*left image*), both oral and pharyngeal chambers are maxed due to the antiresonances in the mouth (oral).

/m/ as in <u>M</u>on<u>u</u>m<u>e</u>nt

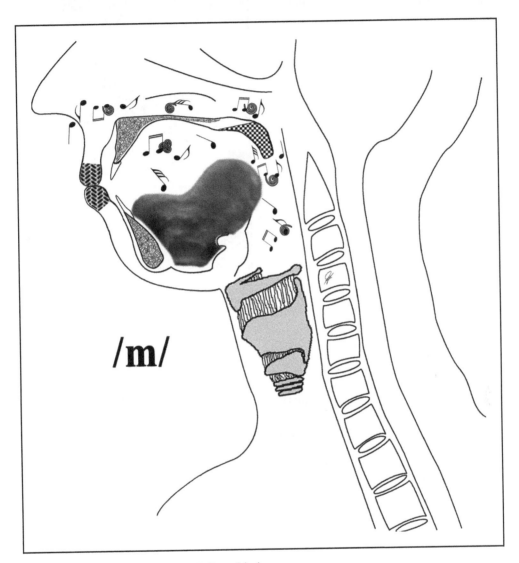

/m/

Figure 8–2. Ultrasound representation of /m/.

Articulatory Considerations

1. Physiological description
   a. The lips are brought together to center, sealing the mouth and with jaw down.
   b. The velopharyngeal port is open.
   c. The tongue forms an open relaxed /ɑ/ for maximum resonance.
   d. The vocal folds come together (adducted), hence creating sound.
   e. The airflow, or in this case the sound, travels through the nasal cavity.

2. Step-by-step instructions

First, let us work on applying the second strategy of the low mandible maneuver (LMM) (Chapter 3) by relaxing and opening the back of the jaw while keeping the lips together to center.

- Close your mouth and put your fingers on the joint that connects the jaw to your skull (temporomandibular joint [TMJ]). You can find that hinge in front of each ear (Chapter 2, Figure 2–5).
- Without pushing it, drop the jaw as far as you can. Keep the lips closed, and feel in your fingers how the bone (condyle) moves forward and bulges. Your larynx will also relax downward.
- Bring the jaw back up and repeat the previous steps to make the movement smoother with each time. Ease the jaw drop by imagining a warm towel on your joint, letting go of tension, and expand the muscles around (masseter and temporalis, Chapter 2, Figure 2–9) and within the joint. Also, keep the muscle around the lips (the orbicularis oris muscle) as loose as possible. Observe if you may have some tension in your cheeks. If you become too tense, reset with some exaggerated chewing motions and massaging your cheeks and TMJ with your hand.

Next, we focus on the tongue.

- Get in front of a mirror or use the reverse camera of your cell phone, drop your jaw without pushing, and say a nice open /ɑ/ as in law.
- See if you can get a little groove in the front part (behind the tip of the tongue) (Figure 8–3) and add a comfortable pitch to it. Have a look at the tongue anatomy picture in the preamble to Part II and imagine the genioglossus

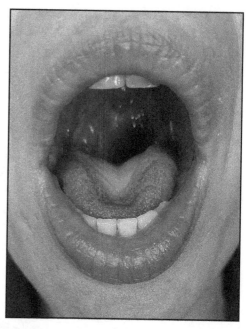

Figure 8–3. The groove behind the tip of the tongue.

depressing downward while expanding the hyoglossus.

- Sustain on the pitch, maintain the tongue shape, and close your lips with the previously acquired drop of the jaw in the back (Figure 8–4). Do you feel a vibration on the tongue surface behind the tongue tip (apex)? If so, this is a good indicator that you created a little groove and increased the oral chamber, creating more CR for the /m/. A good image to keep the tongue shape and front groove, respectively, is to imagine a little scoop of ice cream melting on the front of the tongue, and you do not want the ice cream to touch the teeth around it. You can also put your fingers under your chin and imagine relaxing the big fan-like tongue muscle (genioglossus, Chapter 2, Figure 2–7) down toward your fingers.
- Switch between groove and no groove, dropped and not dropped back of the

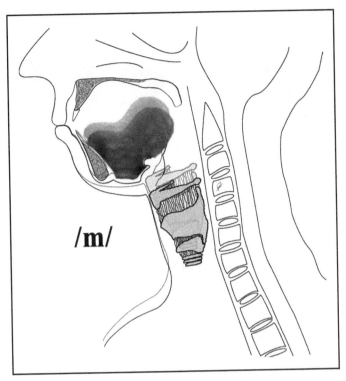

/m/

Figure 8–4. Increasing consonant resonance (CR) by dropping the back of the jaw (see Strategies of the Low Mandible Maneuver, Chapter 3).

jaw, and notice the changes in the vibration and openness. If you get to a good CR, you will feel a vibration (which are the reflections of your sound within the oral cavity) on the tongue surface, the front of the hard palate (alveolar ridge), and your teeth.

Common Challenges

The lips are brought together in order to seal the mouth. However, it is not uncommon to see the lips either pressed together or even sucked in (Figure 8–5). Remember, to ensure maximum CR, we want our two chambers, the mouth and throat (oropharyngeal cavities), to be as relaxed open as possible in order to avoid antiresonances.

To accomplish this, an overexaggeration of lip closure can be observed because the independent control of lips, tongue, jaw, and larynx is not yet established. The challenge is to close the mouth and simultaneously relax the back (posterior) part of the jaw (see the second strategy of the LMM, Chapter 3) as well as the larynx. It seems to provoke a similar instinct as when one pushes against a wall with their hands in order to help arch one's back. The pressed lips serve as a wall, creating a fixed anchor to push the jaw and larynx down from. Unfortunately, it only creates more tension and does not accomplish a relaxed drop of the back of the jaw. Keep the lips loose together and focus on the elongation/expansion of the chewing muscle along the jaw (masseter muscle, Chapter 2, Figure 2–9). Sometimes, it helps

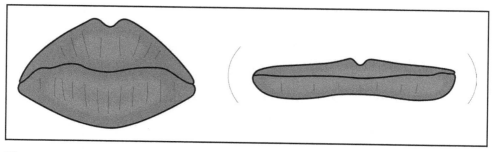

Figure 8–5. Relaxed lip closure (*left*) versus pressed as well as sucked-in lips (*right*).

to imagine putting on a warm towel in this area; it eases every tension and triggers the sensation of relaxation (similar to that which you might feel when you get a facial massage where a warm towel is placed over your face to maintain your relaxed state).

The tongue is another troublemaker, if you will. One way to ensure CR behind the /m/ is to set the preceding or following vowel of the nasal phoneme. However, the /ɑ/ (as in l<u>a</u>w) is a good universal vowel to get maximum CR. Keep in mind, though, that concomitant with a lowered jaw, we have to be more active and pronounced in the tongue movement and shape, respectively. This is another challenge, because in speech we tend not only to be very lazy with our jaw opening but also almost dismissive of any involvement of the tongue. Since we do not have a place of articulation (PoA) for the tongue, phoneticians are susceptible to declare the tongue position as not relevant for /m/. However, as shown over and over throughout the book, this is not true if an actor or singer needs to ensure good projection.

/n/ as in <u>N</u>ick<u>n</u>ame

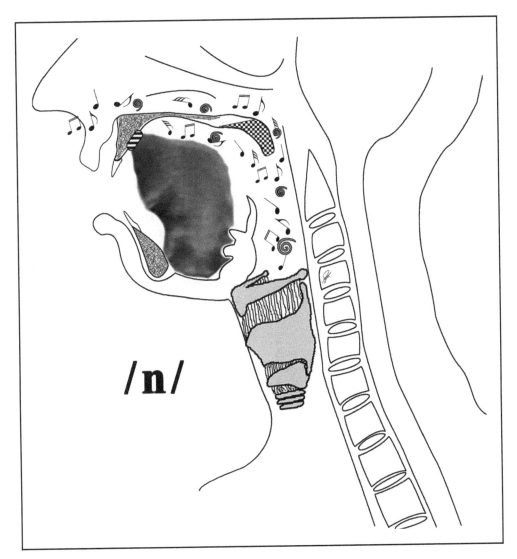

Figure 8–6. Ultrasound representation of /n/.

Articulatory Considerations

1. Physiological description
   a. The lips are neutral and apart.
   b. The velopharyngeal port is open.
   c. The front and the sides of the tongue contact the upper gum ridge.
   d. The vocal folds come together (adducted), hence creating sound.

e. The airflow, or in this case the sound, travels through the nasal cavity.

2. Step-by-step instructions

For the production of /n/, we have to make sure that the tongue seals the oral cavity starting from the front at the alveolar ridge. But first, work on maintaining contact with the tip of the tongue, while dropping the jaw.

■ With the tip of the tongue, establish contact with the roof of the mouth near your upper teeth.
■ Keep the contact and without pushing it, drop the jaw similar to what we have done in the /m/. Only now, you can drop the entire platform (see the first strategy LMM, Chapter 3), not only the back (posterior) part.

Does the tension in your tongue increase when you drop the jaw? This is very common. This is why we need to find the place of articulation (PoA) most suited for our tongue. Why am I saying that? Remember that we all have different shapes and particularly lengths of the tongue. And as we continue to encounter in singing or good speech, it is not just one size fits all. So, to accomplish maximum CR, we need to find the PoA that does not put additional tension in the tongue when trying to keep the mouth open and relaxed.

■ Generally speaking, the PoA (where the tongue touches the roof of the mouth) is the alveolar ridge (gum ridge above your upper teeth). This is particularly true when we do not open our mouth much and the entire tongue does not need to move. However, when we drop the jaw, it increases the distance to the tongue and changes the angle to the tip of the tongue. Thus, we need to find the ideal spot for our tongue that accommodates those changes by sliding along the hard palate (Figure 8–7).
■ Once you have found it, tune in again into the back of the tongue. Have a look at the tongue anatomy pictures (in the preamble to Part II) and imagine letting go of the genioglossus (particularly the

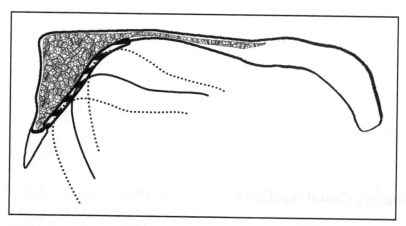

Figure 8–7. Moving along the alveolar ridge to find the ideal place of articulation (PoA) for your tongue while keeping a relaxed, dropped jaw to ensure maximum consonant resonance (CR).

middle and posterior part) as well as the hyoglossus and palatoglossus and feel if that makes maintaining contact while opening your mouth easier. Also, because the palatoglossus is closely associated with the soft palate in function and innervation, imagine the side walls going down from the uvula (palatine aponeurosis turning into the palatoglossus, Figure 8–8) elongate/ expand, subsequently releasing the back

of the tongue (something we naturally do when starting a yawn).

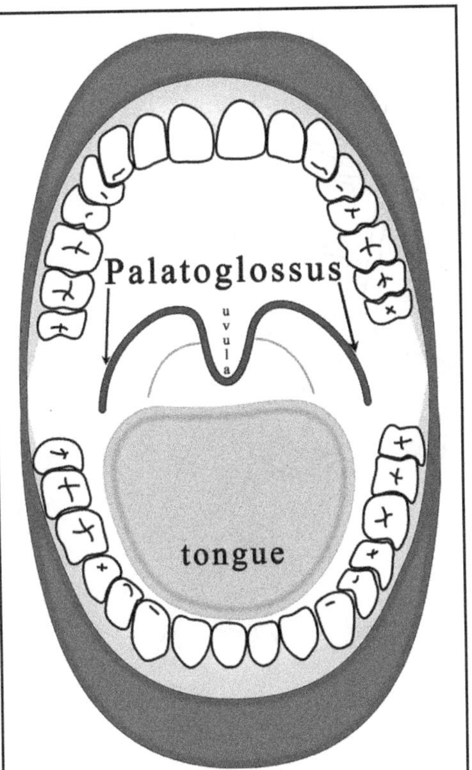

Common Challenges

In this consovowel (pitch + noise, as described in Chapter 7), it is not uncommon to find a push from the root/back of the tongue and larynx in order to establish the PoA (tip of the tongue and gum ridge). It creates an increased sensation that further puts the focus to the front. To help reduce this tendency, it helps to imagine the vowel /ɑ/ (as in l<u>a</u>w). The image relaxes and elongates particularly the root of the tongue as well as the palatoglossus (see Figure 8–8). This increases the pharyngeal cavity, which in turn increases the CR.

In addition, the golden rule of "let physics work for you" (see the preamble to Part II) further prevents the forward push. The sound traveling through the nasal cavity is already enough to ensure the necessary nasality for the phoneme. We do not need to "add" any more by increasing the push against the gum ridge. Once the tongue seals off the oral cavity, it is sealed. This would be like closing a door and then continuing to push, even though it is already closed. Once the filter (tongue, jaw, etc.) is set, notice the increased vibrations (which are the reflections from the sound) in the PoA and possibly along the midline of the tongue surface, while opening up the back (relaxed, elongated tongue root, palatoglossus). This will help you to decouple the source (vibrating vocal folds) from the filter (tongue, jaw, etc.) and ensure maximum CR.

Figure 8–8. Following the side walls and downward from the uvula raises the palatoglossus that inserts into the side of the tongue.

/ŋ/ as in Singing

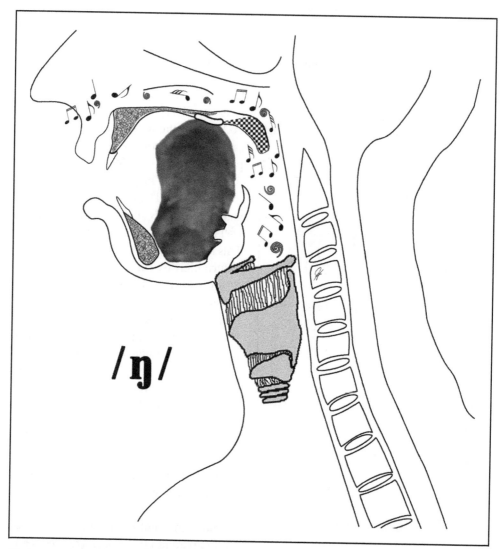

Figure 8–9. Ultrasound representation of /ŋ/.

Articulatory Considerations

1. Physiological description
   a. The lips are neutral and apart.
   b. Tongue body (more toward blade) is raised to contact the soft palate (velum).
   c. The velopharyngeal port is open.
   d. Sides of the center/back tongue contact molars, and back (posterior) upper gum ridge.
   e. The vocal folds come together (adducted), hence creating sound.

f. The airflow, or in this case the sound, travels through the nasal cavity.

2. Step-by-step instructions

The PoA of the nasal consonant may be a bit more challenging, since we have to create it with an open, relaxed mouth while sealing the airflow through the tongue. But, we take one step at the time. First,

■ With your mouth still closed, find contact with the tongue surface (blade, see image in the preamble to Part II) on your hard palate. Also, feel how the sides of your tongue touch the molars, hence sealing the entire mouth. However, it does not necessarily have to touch the molars.

■ Put your fingers on the joint that connects the jaw to your skull (TMJ). You can find that hinge in front of each ear (Chapter 2, Figure 2–5).

■ Without pushing it, drop the jaw as far as you can in a relaxed manner and feel in your fingers how the bone (condyle) moves forward and bulges (LMM, Strategy, Chapter 3). Your larynx will also relax downward.

Now direct your attention to your tongue.

■ Allow the back of the tongue to relax (downward) as well, which serves to elongate its trunk (see the ultrasound image presented earlier).

■ Move the blade along the hard palate and find the PoA that makes the relaxation/drop of the trunk/back of the tongue and jaw easier (Figure 8–10). Remember, this may move farther back (transition of soft/hard palate) than in a regular, jaw-closed speech position.

■ Feel the contact of the tongue surface to the hard palate, imagine letting go of

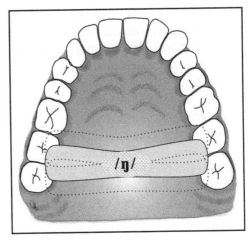

Figure 8–10. Possible places of articulation (PoA) for /ŋ/. Turbulence after release (woven pattern).

any tension in the trunk of the tongue and allow it to elongate (see ultrasound image) while the tip simultaneously retracts.

■ If you are still feeling a lot of tension, reset (circling the jaw, massage the muscles). But before you start again, bite on the edges of your tongue so you can imagine releasing those edges when you set the PoA again.

■ When you are set again, sustain on a pitch and feel the vibration right at the PoA, along the side walls going down from the uvula (palatine aponeurosis turning into the palatoglossus, see Figure 8–8) and the center of the hard palate. Imagine the vibration to reflect back into the throat (pharynx) to avoid constriction and forward pushing in and from the larynx/tongue.

Common Challenges

Finding the right PoA may be the biggest challenge in this consovowel (pitch + noise; Chapter 7). In speech without CR, we only move the back/root of the tongue upward to establish contact with the palate. However, with the LMM (relaxed, dropped jaw), we are increasing the oral distance; hence, the root of the tongue needs to elongate. Therefore, it is no longer the body of the tongue that establishes contact with the PoA. Also, remember to find your vertically most comfortable PoA. As indicated in Figure 8–10, this can be in the vicinity of the transition of hard to soft palate and most likely will move a bit backward, once you open up the mouth. Furthermore, the release and elongation of the genioglossus, hyoglossus, palatoglossus (see graphics in the preamble to Part II), as well as the side of the tongue edges are necessary to ease this effort. For the latter, it helps to bite on the edges of your tongue, putting the focus and feeling on them, so you can imagine letting them go (retract). Another aid to help guide the tongue would be a tongue depressor. Remember the exer-

cise in Chapter 4, where we help guide the outward and inward movement of the tongue without curling the tip? By putting the tongue depressor on the tip of the tongue, the necessary retraction for your /ŋ/ (see ultrasound image) will become easier, and you can focus on the elongation of the tongue root.

Another indication of too much stiffness and spreading within the tongue and/or jaw is the vibration on the hard palate as well as those side walls coming down from the uvula and turning into the palatoglossus (palatine aponeurosis, see Figure 8–8). If you feel the vibration more spread to the side instead of centered on the hard palate and barely any vibration in the side walls down the uvula (palatine aponeurosis), it is quite possible that the back of the tongue and the lips are spread rather than vertically relaxed and elongated.

/l/ as in <u>L</u>ong

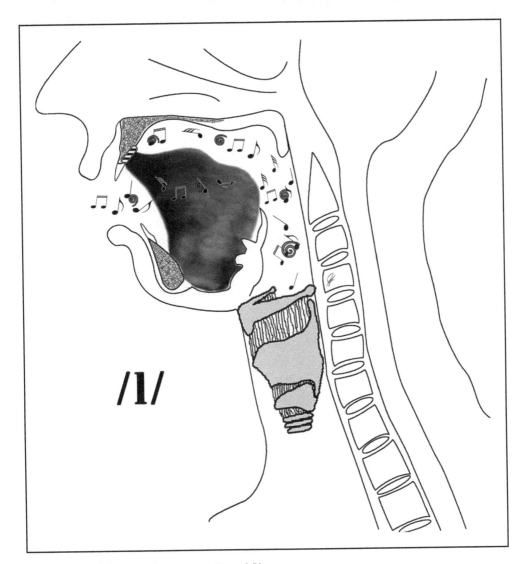

Figure 8–11. Ultrasound representation of /l/.

Articulatory Considerations

1. Physiological description
   a. The lips are neutral and apart.
   b. The tip of the tongue contacts the upper gum ridge.
   c. The velopharyngeal port is closed.
   d. The vocal folds come together (adducted), hence creating sound.
   e. The airflow, or in this case the sound, travels through the oral cavity around the sides of the tongue.

2. Step-by-step instructions

In the consovowel /l/, we find similarities to /n/ in terms of the PoA, except now, the tip of the tongue (apex) does not need to seal the oral cavity. This also why it is called continuants. First though, we have to work again on maintaining contact with the tip of the tongue, while dropping the jaw.

■ With the mouth still closed, establish contact with the tip of the tongue by touching the roof of the mouth near your upper teeth.

■ Keep the contact and without pushing it, drop the jaw similar to what we have done in /m/. Only now, you can drop the entire platform (first strategy LMM, Chapter 3), not only the back (posterior) part.

Does the tension in your tongue increase when you drop the jaw? Again, this is very common. As you recall from the /n/, in order to accomplish maximum CR, we need to find the PoA most suited for our tongue because of its individual size and length. By doing so, we are able to relax all active articulators and more particularly not put additional tension in the back of the tongue when trying to keep the mouth open and relaxed.

■ Generally speaking, the PoA (where the tongue touches the roof of the mouth) is the alveolar ridge (gum ridge above your upper teeth). This is particularly true when we do not open our mouth much and the entire tongue does not need to move much. However, when we drop the jaw, it increases the distance to the tongue and changes the angle to the tip of the tongue. Thus, we need to find the ideal spot for our tongue that accommodates those changes by sliding along the hard palate (see Figure 8–7).

■ Once you have found it, tune in again into the back of the tongue. Have a look at the tongue anatomy pictures and imagine letting go of the genioglossus (particularly the middle and posterior part) as well as the hyoglossus and palatoglossus and feel if that makes maintaining contact while opening your mouth easier. Also, imagine the side walls going down from the uvula (palatine aponeurosis turning into the palatoglossus, see Figure 8–8) elongate/expand, subsequently releasing the back of the tongue.

■ On a pitch, start phonating the consovowel /l/ and imagine an open vowel, such as /ɑ/, around it. Notice the vibrations (which are the reflections of the sound within the oral cavity) at the PoA (alveolar ridge), on the surface and the edges of the tongue, and possibly even the lower teeth.

Common Challenges

With the sound moving around the sides of the tongue (Figure 8–12), we have to make sure the tongue does not spread, particularly in the back. It will not only make it physically uncomfortable but also give the /l/ (as in long) a more velar (soft palate) like quality (as in silk). Remember the source-filter theory (Chapter 5), where the source sound (vibrating vocal folds) changes with every adjustment of the filter (tongue, jaw, etc.). Moving the body of the tongue in the vicinity of the soft palate changes not only the shape of the tongue but subsequently the vocal tract as well. The influence of the phonetic environment is of course a major contributor to this change for both native and non-native speakers of American English (Edwards, 2003). In our example, "silk," it is the /k/ following the /l/. Try it out. Exe-

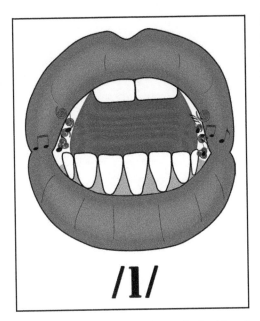

/ l /

Figure 8–12. Sound passing on both sides of the tongue (front [coronal] view).

cuting each phoneme, say the word "silk" very slowly. Take notice what the back of the tongue is doing when you sustain on the /l/. Can you feel a little spread and upward push from the back of the tongue? This is because the tongue is already preparing for the /k/,

like a coarticulation (Chapter 9). Of course, it may not be avoidable completely, though the degree on how much can be tolerated in terms of idiomacy and CR ought to be on the radar. Our goal as singers and actors is to reduce the influence of the phonetic environment as well as the transition from phoneme to phoneme to an unnoticeable minimum.

To help reduce the tendency to spread the back of the tongue and consequently stiffen the larynx, it helps to imagine the vowel /ɑ/ (as in l<u>aw</u>). Because of the necessary contact in the front (tip of the tongue and gum ridge), this often results in a push from the tongue root, the larynx, or both. The image of the vowel /ɑ/ relaxes and elongates the root of the tongue, the edges, as well as the palatoglossus (see Figure 8–9), increasing the pharyngeal cavity. This in turn increases the CR and reduces the degree of the velar-like quality. However, if a characterization of a role asks for it, we may even want to exaggerate the /k/ approximation to the soft palate, though not by initiation with a push from the larynx (see Chapter 9, stop consonants).

9 Stop Consonants—/p/ /t/ /k/

As the word implies, these noises, or aspirations, are made with a complete blockage of airflow, creating a pressure chamber, followed by a release of that air. This is why they are also referred to as plosives. But why am I saying "noises"? Because the vocal folds are not together (abducted), no sound is coming out. It is the burst of air, the audible friction after the release of the blockage that creates turbulence, which in turn creates the noise associated with the particular phoneme. Of course, we could use the term *sound,* but then we would need to add the word *aperiodic,* which is the nature of "noise" because the pattern does not repeat itself. Periodic sounds, on the other hand, are where the pattern repeats itself, and they are rich in harmonics. This is an oversimplification of fundamental acoustics, and I refer everyone who wants to get deeper into that subject to Titze's *Principles of Voice Production* (2000). For the sake of simplicity, we use *sound* when there is actually a pitch, and *noise* when there is only friction through air.

Now, if there is only noise, how are we able to distinguish between the various noises of /p/, /k/, and /t/? For that we have to remind ourselves of the source-filter theory (discussed in Chapter 5). Any changes in the vocal tract (tongue, jaw, lips,

and combinations of them) are filtering the source (sound) coming from the vocal folds. Although in this case we do not have sound coming, the same is true with breath streams. In our stop consonants, each place of articulation (PoA) is blocking the air either with the lips (labial, for /p/), the teeth and/or gum ridge (alveolar, for /t/), or the tongue on the soft palate (velar, for /k/). Thus, air pressure is building up right behind those places, and the turbulence creates different frictions after their release. For instance, the lips have a soft surface, which means that any airstream passing through them will not have as much constriction and friction as when passing through the teeth. With the latter, the airstream for /t/ (as in tiny) is a diffused friction on a hard surface, generating a much more strident noise than the released air pressure for /p/ (as in pizza).

Because we are only dealing with air to create pressure chambers, we also have to deal with the aftermath of the turbulence (Figure 9–1). After the release of the constriction, there is a decrease in pressure within the constriction. Hence, there is no longer an outward force on the wall of the constriction (palate and tongue surface), and it will begin to return to the position it would have in the absence of intraoral pressure.

For this reason, one of the critical parts in the production of consonants is the transition from the consonant to the vowel. It

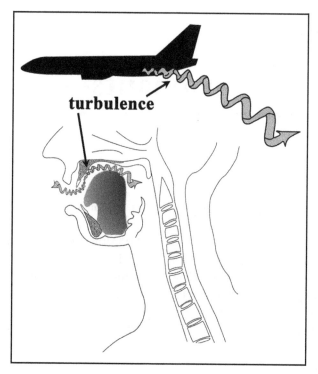

Figure 9–1. Turbulence after the release of the stop consonant /t/.

is crucial to keep the time from the release of the stop consonant to the start of the vowel (also called voice onset time [VOT]) as seamless and clean as possible. Think of airplanes at takeoff. When an airplane takes off, the turbulence generated necessitates the next in line waiting until the turbulent air is cleared. Failure to do so could cause that plane to turn over, especially if it is smaller than the preceding one. Similarly, after any stop consonant, we ought to anticipate the change in pressure by continuing the support (preventing collapse within the vocal tract and rib cage, as well as exact maneuvering of articulators) and give a little room before the following vowel. On the spectrogram you can actually see a gap spanning milliseconds (little more than a tenth of a second) that not only gives the tongue the

time to shape and set the vowel but also the burst of air to settle down before the actual phonation begins (Figure 9–2). If we do not make that clean transition, we experience coarticulation, which affects the vowel and weakens the consonants. We go through a meticulous practice process in our first stop consonants.

Finally, a comparison of the ultrasound images of the stop consonants with the prevoiced stop consonants (Chapter 10) shows the significant effect of the increase of intraoral pressure. This is particularly true for the displacement of the tongue root, increasing the pharyngeal volume due to the passive response to the pressure increase. In addition, there may also be an active response from the fibers of the posterior genioglossus muscles (Stevens, 2000).

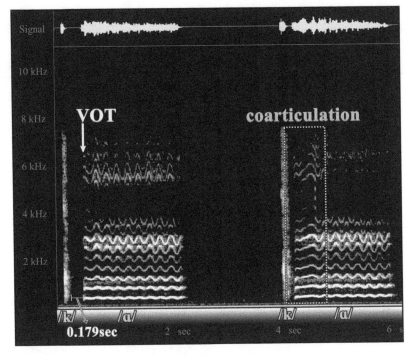

Figure 9–2. Clean transition between /k/ and /ɑ/ (*left*). Turbulence after the release of the stop consonant /k/ affecting the following vowel.

/p/ as in Pizza

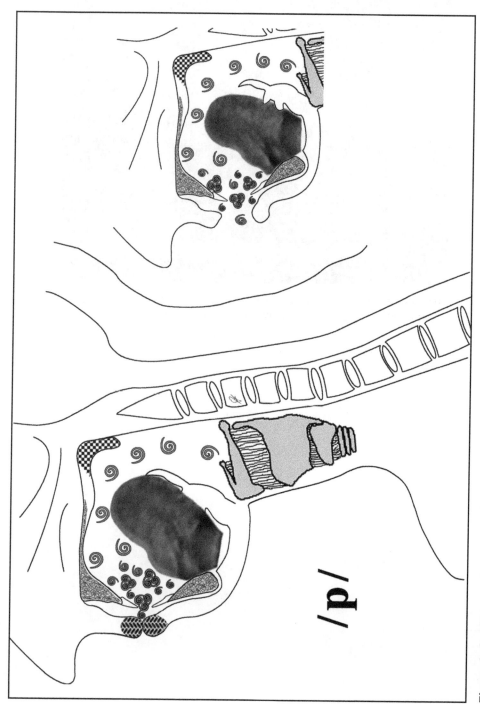

Figure 9–3. Ultrasound representation of /p/.

Articulatory Considerations

1. Physiological description
   a. The lips are brought together.
   b. The tongue position should give room to both chambers, mouth (oral), and throat (pharyngeal) to balance the increased pressure (may be similar to an /a/ vowel).
   c. The velopharyngeal port is closed.
   d. The vocal folds are not together (abducted); hence, there is no sound.
   e. The air pressure is building up behind the lips.
   f. Once the lips part, the turbulence (airflow around the lips) creates the noise associated with the phoneme.

2. Step-by-step instructions

In order to sensitize ourselves to the stop-action of the plosives, we start by exploring what it feels like when pressure increases inside our mouth (oral cavity), nose (nasal cavity), and throat (pharyngeal cavity).

- Take a breath, then close your mouth and nose (pinch it with your fingers) and try to push out air while keeping everything closed. Can you feel an airwave traveling along your vocal tract and pushing against your lips (possibly puffing out your cheeks like a squirrel collecting hazelnuts) and nose?
- Continue with two to three pulses at a time from your lower abdomen to feel the air particles traveling forward like a wave, only now we cannot see it and merely feel.
- Next, try to repeat the same without pinching your nose, instead closing the path to the nose through the uvula (velopharyngeal port). It is like learning how to dive without pinching your nose. Should you have trouble with this,

have a look at the Common Challenges section presented later for some help.
- Continue the exercise and start including a relaxed tongue by imagining an /a/ (as in law) behind it. That will give you the groove in the front that will help you to both balance the pressure turbulence after the release and secure a wider and cleaner frequency spectrum (high and low as well as less-scattered formants). You may feel how the pressure pushes on your tongue surface because of the pushback once it hit the teeth.
- Finally, prepare a good pressure buildup and release it without losing the energy by collapsing your rib cage or closing the jaw. Imagine the direction of the "explosion" to go back into your mouth instead of outward. That will help you to balance out the sudden pressure changes and turbulence and not lose or even push the "explosion" outward by engaging your larynx.

Common Challenge

Similar to the /m/ consonant (Chapter 8), we do not want to press, spread, and/or suck in the lips to counteract the increase in pressure (Figure 9–4). They may be a bit puckered but minimally. Also, watch out for puffed-up cheeks because that is an indicator that the airstream is just randomly moving wherever there is an opening or less resistance. In order to avoid having this energy spread to the side, give a little direction with your cheek by engaging the corner of your mouth. If you have ever played a woodwind instrument (e.g., flute), you will remember how you guided the air through a little hole in the center of your lips. If not, imagine you have some water in

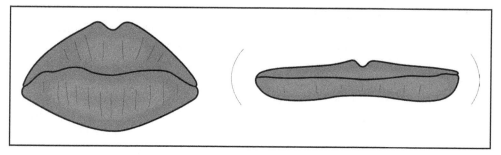

Figure 9–4. Relaxed, puckered lips (*left*) versus spread lips (*right*).

your mouth that you want to spray out like a fountain stream, guiding the stream into the center by sealing the corners of your mouth, which in turn engages your cheeks as well. This will make the lips a little stiffer and therefore not puff out. But as always, it is the balance between tension and active engagement that we are looking for.

Another challenge may be the closure of the velopharyngeal port. Sometimes, the pressure buildup can feel too much for some. So, keeping the velopharyngeal port open is like a valve in a pressure cooker, though acoustically, it turns into an /m/ sound rather than a plosive. So how are we going to make that happen? That is a good question. The answer might sound way too simple for the complexity of the vocal tract: you just need to think of wanting the uvula to close and it will happen. We have programmed mechanisms that are triggered by signals to and from our brain. For instance, having food in our mouth that is about to be swallowed is the signal to the brain that we are about to pass food along the uvula (closing it), and everything else is set in place to guide it into the esophagus and not the trachea. We are not going to take food in, but we can help by aiding the closure through pinching the nose and learn what it feels like along the soft palate once it closes.

One more factor to consider in all voiceless stops in prevocalic positions is the

delayed voicing of the following vowel relative to the release of the stop. We already mentioned the VOT. However, we have not yet discussed how we can practice it. Here we are taking /p/ as an example on how to practice stop consonants, but the basic concept is the same for all stop consonants.

How, then, do we practice it? Let us assume we have the word /pæk/, as in "pack" (which also gives us a nice /k/ at the end) and use the spectrogram as a biofeedback tool (Figure 9–5). First, we start by executing the stop consonant /p/ and then, after a second or two, follow with the vowel /æ/, as in "and," and after another couple of seconds conclude with /k/. While this gap between the consonants and vowel is too large, it gives you enough time to first focus and concentrate on the execution of /p/ (preparing the pressure buildup, feeling the burst of energy in your mouth after the release and how it spreads around, etc.), set the vowel /æ/ without any tongue shape changes (you will see a clean on-/offset and horizontal lines), and conclude with the /k/ (find PoA, buildup pressure, etc.). This establishes the shape and mechanism for each phoneme so we know where we have to go: start with point A, go to B, and finally to C. Repeat it a couple of times and make sure that the support for the stop consonants comes with an additional impulse from your lower abdominal muscles (under your belly but-

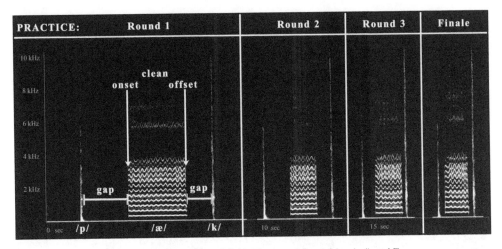

Figure 9–5. Practice protocol for /p/ and /k/ in the word /pæk/ (as in "pack").

ton) instead of the throat, and that the vowel always has a clean start and ending.

Once you think you have found the maximum consonant resonance (CR), you can start to shorten the gap between the consonants and vowel. Give your brain time to learn the new habits and do not speed up too soon. With every acceleration, make sure you maintain the established parameters from the first round for each consonant. If that is not possible, you need to go back to the timing where you were able to do so. The goal is to make the transition between the phonemes as seamless as possible, where the necessary changes of various articulators (tongue, jaw, etc.) need to be well coordinated, so none of them influences or distorts the other phoneme. Think of it like being a robot. If a robot is programmed to open the jaw, it will go from position A, closed, to position B, open, in a matter of milliseconds without any detour. This is exactly what we are practicing: first, knowing the execution of each phoneme and then moving like a robot from /p/ to /æ/ to /k/.

Of course, remember the "say it as a singer" (SAS) meme. The same applies when

we want to achieve maximum CR as actors and actresses (Figure 9–6). Though before continuing, we should discuss the clean transition or offset, respectively, between the vowel and consonant /k/. Unlike in singing, where a single pitch is sustained throughout the vowel, in the spoken word the inflection (pitch) within a vowel will descend. Thus, the lines will not stay completely horizontal and show a little downward movement at the end of the vowel. However, the offset should still look clean cut, maintaining a little gap after it.

Let us conclude with one more challenge that will be seen in almost all of the voiceless and prevoiced consonants. More often than not, tension in the larynx will emanate in order to "create" the noise part of the consonant. In this case, I always say, "Let physics work for you." The release of the tongue contact to another surface (teeth, palate) is creating the noise part associated with the consonant. Hence, there is no need to separately add any muscular action by pushing harder, particularly not from the throat. The image of picturing the explosion going backward into the mouth helps to prevent that particular constriction in the larynx.

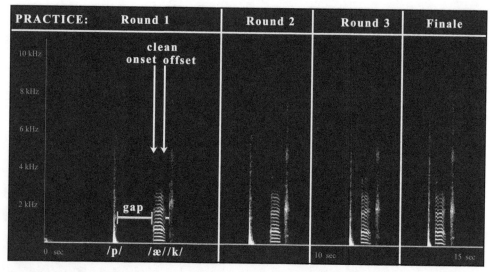

Figure 9–6. Practice protocol for /p/ and /k/ in the word /pæk/ (as in "pack").

/t/ as in <u>T</u>ime

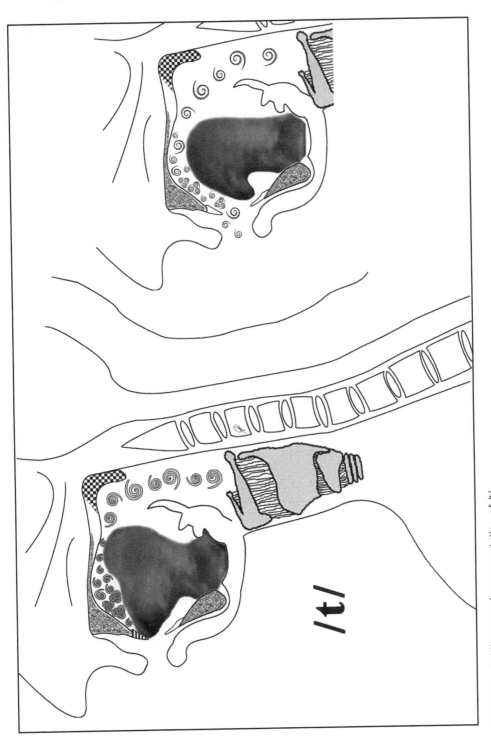

Figure 9–7. Ultrasound representation of /t/.

Articulatory Considerations

1. Physiological description
   a. The lips are apart though a little protruded (like a tube).
   b. The mandible is lowered slightly in back (low mandible maneuver [LMM], second strategy).
   c. The tongue tip contacts the teeth, and the tongue sides contact the upper gum (alveolar) ridge in the front (anteriorly) and the sides (laterally).
   d. The velopharyngeal port is closed.
   e. The air pressure is building up behind the gum ridge and teeth.
   f. Once the tongue releases the contact, the turbulence (air along the hard palate, teeth, and tongue surface) creates the noise associated with the phoneme.

2. Step-by-step instructions

The main articulator for this consonant is the tongue.

■ With the mouth comfortably open, make contact with the tip of the tongue behind the upper teeth. The tongue sides should be sealed along the upper gum ridge (Figure 9–8).

■ The lips may be a little protruded, like a tube, which will prevent them from spreading but also help balance out the turbulence and pressure changes after the release (Figure 9–9).

■ Prepare a good pressure buildup, possibly feel a little groove (like an air bolus right behind the tip of the tongue)

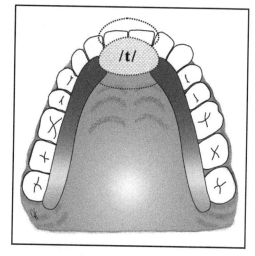

Figure 9–8. Tip of the tongue's possible places of articulation (PoA) for /t/. Turbulence (woven pattern) after anterior release of the tongue tip.

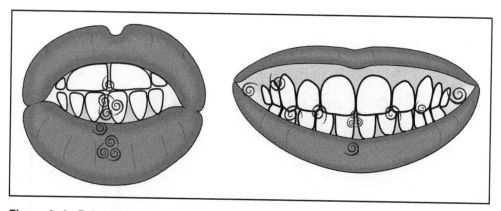

Figure 9–9. Relaxed, puckered lips (*left*) versus spread lips (*right*).

and release it without losing the energy by collapsing your rib cage or closing the jaw. The opening of the closure should start at the center behind the teeth; thus, the constriction and turbulence should also be felt and maintained right there (see Figure 9–6) and not spread to the sides. To prevent tension, imagine the direction of the "explosion" going backward into your mouth instead of outward. This will help you to balance out the pressure changes and turbulence and not lose the "explosion" or push it outward, by engaging your larynx and collapsing your rib cage.

■ After the pressure release, you may also feel reflections from the teeth on the tongue surface.

Common Challenges

Finding the right spot for the PoA is also a common challenge for this consonant. Generally, the tip of the tongue will be behind the upper teeth. However, should you have a long tongue or possibly want more of the almost harsh burst, you might have the PoA in the middle of both upper and lower teeth and seal off with the blade and sides of the tongue starting from the alveolar ridge. This will, once you release, give you even more hard surface (both upper and lower teeth) to reflect on. If you want the opposite, you might want to move the PoA up to the alveolar ridge. Of course, let us not forget the context of the following vowel or consonant (e.g., /ts/ as in ca<u>ts</u>) that will also influence that decision.

Spreading the lips as an instinctive counteraction to the increase in pressure is also likely to occur. The lips rounding in combination with the tongue groove will help funnel the airstream with all its energy to the center of the teeth and not spread it to the side, losing the power. Concomitant with that, tension emanates in the larynx in order to "create" the noise part of the consonant. As suggested before, "let physics work for you." The release of the tongue contact to the palate is creating the noise part associated with the consonant. Hence, there is no need to separately add any muscular action by pushing harder, particularly not from the throat. Feel the backpressure (e.g., in the back of the soft palate, groove in the front of the tongue, etc.) once you start the pressurization. On release, imagine the explosion going backward into the mouth to prevent the constriction in the larynx.

/k/ as in Communication

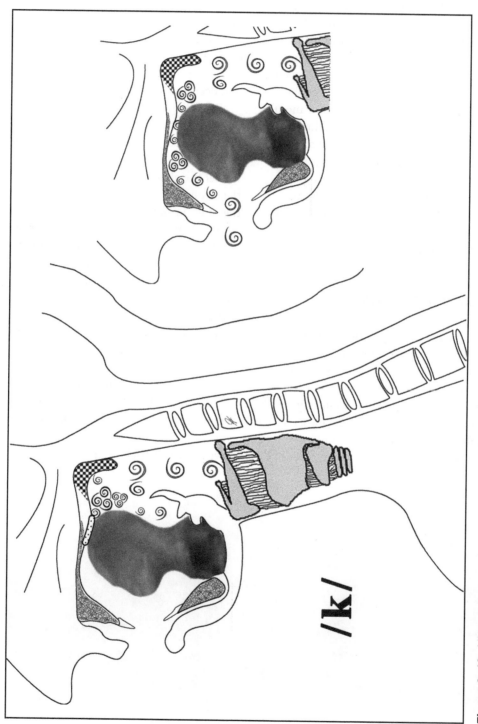

Figure 9–10. Ultrasound representation of /k/.

Articulatory Considerations

1. Physiological description
   a. The lips are apart and neutral.
   b. The tongue body is raised to create a seal across the soft palate, back molars, and the back (posterior) gum ridge.
   c. The velopharyngeal port is closed.
   d. The vocal folds are not together (abducted), hence no sound.
   e. The air pressure is building up behind the tongue and soft palate seal.
   f. Once the tongue releases the contact, the turbulence (air along the hard palate and tongue surface) creates the noise associated with the phoneme.

2. Step-by-step instructions

The stop action of this plosive may be a bit more challenging, since we have to create it with an open, relaxed mouth while sealing the airflow through the tongue. But one step at a time.

- With your mouth still closed, find contact with the tongue surface (blade) on your hard palate. Also, feel how the sides of your tongue touch the molars, hence sealing the entire mouth.
- Put your fingers on the joint that connects the jaw to your skull (temporomandibular joint). You can find that hinge in front of each ear, as described in Chapter 2, Figure 2–5.
- Without pushing it, drop the jaw as far as you can in a relaxed manner, and with your fingers, feel how the bone (condyle) moves forward and bulges. Your larynx will also relax downward.

Now place your attention on your tongue.

- Allow the back of the tongue to relax (downward) as well, so it can elongate its root (see the ultrasound image presented earlier).
- Move the blade of your tongue along the hard palate and find the spot (PoA) that makes the relaxation/drop of the root/back of the tongue and jaw easier (Figure 9–11).

Feel the contact of the tongue surface to the hard palate, imagine letting go of any tension in the trunk of the tongue, and allow it to elongate (see ultrasound image).

- If you are still feeling a lot of tension, reset. But before you start again, bite on the edges of your tongue, and once you set the PoA again, imagine releasing those edges.
- Once you are set again, allow for a good pressure buildup and release it without losing the energy by collapsing your rib cage or closing the jaw. The opening of the closure should start at the center; thus, the constriction and turbulence should also be felt and maintained right

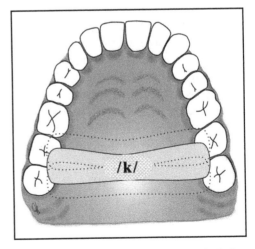

Figure 9–11. Possible places of articulation (PoA) for /k/. Turbulence after release (woven pattern).

there (Figure 9–8) and not spread to the sides. As with both /p/ and /t/, imagine the direction of the "explosion" going back down to your throat instead of outward. This will help you to balance out the pressure changes and turbulence and not lose or even push the "explosion" outward by engaging your larynx.

Common Challenges

Possibly the biggest challenge with this consonant is finding the right PoA. In speech without CR, we only move the back/root of the tongue upward to establish contact with the palate. However, with the relaxed, dropped jaw, we are increasing the oral distance; hence, the root of tongue needs to elongate, and therefore, it is no longer the articulator that establishes contact with the PoA. Also, remember to find your most comfortable vertical PoA. As indicated in Figure 9–8, this can be in the vicinity of the transition of hard to soft palate and most likely will move backward a little once you open up your mouth. Furthermore, the release and elongation of the genioglossus, hyoglossus, palatoglossus (see the graphics in the preamble to Part II) as well as the side of the tongue edges are necessary to relieve this effort. For the latter, it again helps to bite on the edges of your tongue, placing your focus and feeling on them, so you can imagine letting them go (retracting).

Tension in the larynx in order to "create" the noise part of the consonant may also occur. Once again, let physics work for you. As with any of the stop consonants, the release of the tongue contact to the palate is creating the noise part associated with the consonant. Hence, there is no need to add any additional push, particularly not from the throat. The image of picturing an explosion going backward into the mouth prevents constriction in the larynx.

Should you practice with a spectrogram, you want to watch out for higher and lower frequencies to assure maximum CR. Remember the "two chambers" connected through a "hallway" concept from Chapters 5, 7, and 8? If the room in the front is too small either because of the missing groove in the tongue or the LMM, we are creating antiresonances that cancel out the lower frequencies. In Figure 9–12, you can see the two chambers are set with maximum space (left, gray/red). Once the release of the stop consonant occurs, the air particles have room to reflect front and back. On the other side (right, tiles/green), the front chamber does not provide enough room. Thus, with the release, the higher frequencies are not going to be amplified by the lower ones and will likely disappear in larger and poor acoustic theaters and concert halls. Remember, we are always showing the maximum CR. Hence, actors may not always have their jaw droppped as far using the second strategy of the LMM (Chapter 3). However, the tip of the tongue is still more retracted and the back/root of the tongue elongated in order to leave more room in the front.

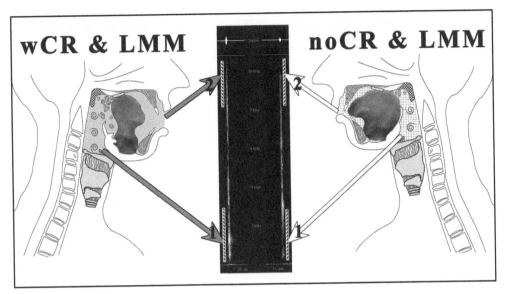

Figure 9–12. Setup of the phoneme /ç/ before the release. On the left (*gray/red*) with maximum consonant resonance and low mandible maneuver and on the right without (*tiles/green*). Note the difference in higher and lower frequencies as well as the intensity (signal).

References

Stevens, K.N., (2000) *Acoustic phonetics.* Cambridge, MA: MIT Press.

Titze, I. (2000). *Principles of voice production* (2nd ed.). Iowa City, IA: National Center for Voice and Speech.

10 Prevoiced Stop Consonants—/b/ /d/ /g/

General Considerations

In the previous chapter, we discussed those stop consonants that have no pitch component and hence are voiceless. Each of those consonants is homorganic with our prevoiced stop consonant /b, d, g/. The particular order represents the same place of articulation front to back, where the full occlusion of the oral airway occurs (remember, the velopharyngeal port [uvula] is closed as well). These consonants also require an accumulation of pressure whose acute release creates the noise part associated with the consonant. So far, sounds pretty familiar, right? However, now, before the release of the built-up pressure, we also have to add a pitch/sound component.

How do we do that without any opening? We couple it with the pressurization because this is the only time when air is moving through the vocal folds. Thus, the airflow sets the folds into vibration, creating this millisecond of a sound. Let us do a funny test together. On a comfortable pitch, sustain on an /m/ (as in mountain), and with your fingers, abruptly close your nose.

Did you notice the very short continuation of the pitch after you closed off the nasal cavity? You can also try to close both mouth and nose and then start phonating an /m/. Did you hear how short it is and how the pressure simultaneously builds up as well? Of course, we do not want to keep using our hands for help. Remember, the uvula in the back closes with your focus and attention to do so. It is the same as when you jump into the water, only there you feel the invisible membrane between the water and inside pressure in your nose better because of the two different mediums.

The biggest trap in prevoicing is substitution with a nasal consonant. It often happens because of either a lack of awareness when the velopharyngeal port is open or an attempt to exaggerate it for better audibility on stage.

In the spectrogram, we can clearly see the differences (Figure 10–1). We ought to be careful not to do so, since the audience can clearly discern the difference. For that, the spectrogram is a wonderful tool to help monitor and practice the prevoicing. So, let us get right to it.

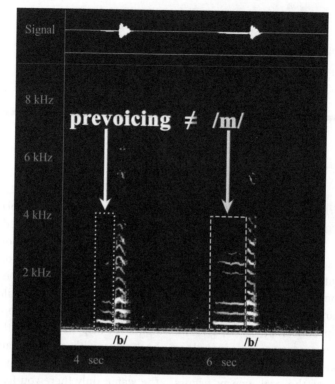

Figure 10–1. Prevoiced (*left*) versus nasal (*right*).

/b/ as in Bubble

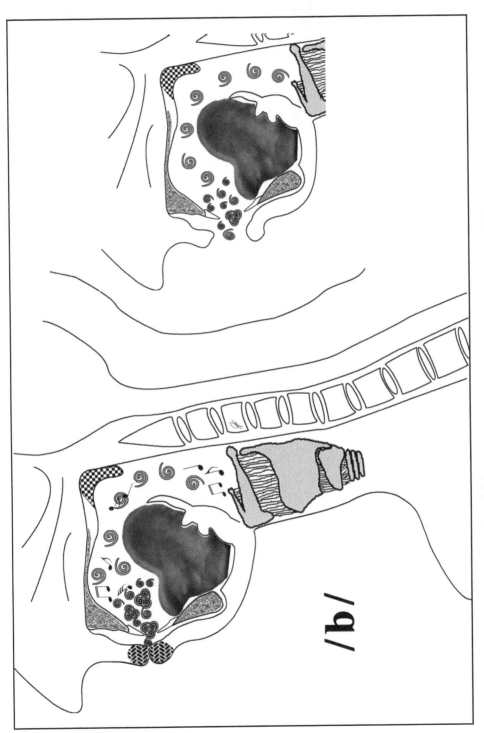

Figure 10–2. Ultrasound representation of /b/.

Articulatory Considerations

1. Physiological description
   a. The lips are brought together.
   b. The tongue position should give room to both chambers, mouth (oral), and throat (pharyngeal) to balance the increased pressure (may be similar to an /a/ vowel).
   c. The velopharyngeal port is closed.
   d. The vocal folds come together (adducted), hence creating sound for a brief moment (pitch only for a brief moment in prevoice).
   e. The air pressure is building up behind the lips.
   f. Once the lips part, the turbulence (airflow around the lips) creates the noise associated with the phoneme.

2. Step-by-step instructions

Since prevoiced consonants are homorganic to the stop consonants, much will be similar in their execution. Only now, we are adding sound into the mix. But simple as it might sound, it adds quite another set of challenges. Because the onset of the sound (vocal fold vibration) begins close to the burst, there is little opportunity for an interval of aspiration to occur.

- First, be sure not to overdo this exercise and be gentle with it. Take a breath, then close your mouth and nose (pinch it with your fingers) and try to make a sound while keeping everything closed. Can you hear how short it is? Do you also feel an airwave simultaneously traveling along your vocal tract and pushing against your lips (possibly puffing out your cheeks like a squirrel collecting hazelnuts) and nose?

- Continue this exercise with two to three pulses at a time from your lower abdomen to feel the connection of the sound and air particles traveling forward like a wave.

- Next, try to repeat, without pinching your nose, thus closing the path to the nose through the uvula (velopharyngeal port). It is like learning how to dive without pinching your nose. Should you have trouble with this, revisit the Common Challenges in Chapter 9, p. 165

- Continue the exercise and introduce a relaxed tongue by imagining an /a/ (as in l<u>a</u>w) behind it. That will give you the groove in the front, which in turn will help you to both have maximum resonance for the sound and balance the pressure turbulence after the release. You may feel a vibration on your tongue surface from the sound reflection of the teeth.

- Finally, phonate with a good pressure buildup to the point when it comes to a natural stop, and release it without losing the sound and energy by collapsing your rib cage and/or closing the jaw. Imagine the direction of the release going back into your mouth instead of out. That will help you to balance out the sudden pressure changes and turbulence and support the lower frequencies of the sound spectrum without pushing the "explosion" outward by engaging your larynx.

Common Challenges

Because of the similarities of the basic concept compared to the stop consonants (discussed in Chapter 9), you may already anticipate some of the challenges that might arise. Starting with the lips, we want to watch out for any tension through spreading, sucking into the mouth, or the like, and possibly counterpart it by puckering them a little (Figure 10–3).

Additionally, watch out for puffed-up cheeks. We want to guide the airstream with all its energy to the center of the lips and not spread it to the side, losing the power. It may be helpful, in addition to the first step of the exercise (pinching your nose for the prevoiced part), to also bring in a spectro-gram to help monitor the progress with the help of the nose pinch (see Figure 10–1). In addition, as mentioned earlier, the biggest trap is substituting the prevoiced part with an /m/ instead of the very short voicing preceding the stop release. Using the hands and possibly a spectrograph for monitoring (or recording yourself) will help with sensitizing the difference.

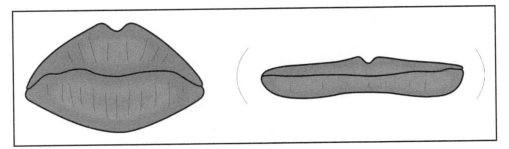

Figure 10–3. Relaxed, puckered lips (*left*) versus spread lips (*right*).

/d/ as in Dog

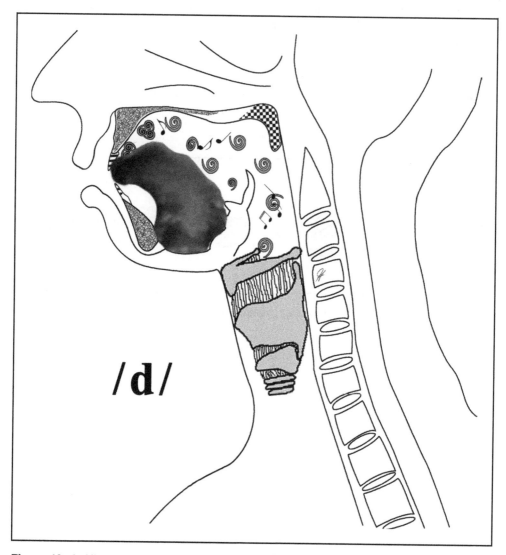

Figure 10–4. Ultrasound representation of /d/.

Articulatory Considerations

1. Physiological description
   a. The lips are apart and slightly protruded (round, like an /o/).
   b. The front and sides of the tongue contact the upper (sometimes also lower) teeth and the upper gum ridge (alveolar) in the front (anteriorly) and along the sides (laterally).
   c. The velopharyngeal port is closed.
   d. The vocal folds come together (adducted), hence creating sound

(pitch) only for a brief moment in prevoicing.

e. The air pressure is building up behind the tongue and alveolar ridge.

f. Once the tongue releases the contact, the sound of the following vowel is released, and the turbulence creates the noise associated with the phoneme.

2. Step-by-step instructions

As with the /t/ (Chapter 9), the main articulator is the tongue.

◼ With the mouth comfortably open, find contact with the tip of the tongue behind the upper teeth. The tongue sides are sealing along the upper gum ridge (Figure 10–5).

◼ The lips may be a little protruded, like a tube, which will prevent them from spreading but also help balance out the turbulence and pressure changes after the release (Figure 10–6).

◼ Finally, phonate with a good pressure buildup to the point when it comes to a natural stop, and release it without losing the sound and energy by closing the jaw and/or collapsing your rib cage. Imagine the direction of the release

going back into your mouth instead of outward. That will help you to balance out the sudden pressure changes and turbulence without pushing the air outward by engaging your larynx.

◼ With the onset of the sound (vocal fold vibration) starting close to the burst, after the pressure release you may also feel some of the sound reflection on the tongue surface (blade in front).

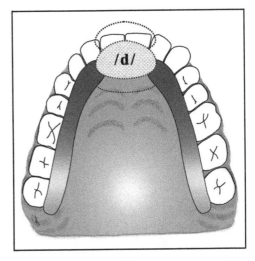

Figure 10–5. Tip of the tongue's possible places of articulation (PoA) for /d/. Turbulence (woven pattern) after anterior release of the tongue tip.

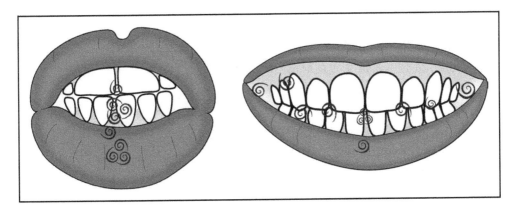

Figure 10–6. Relaxed, puckered lips (*left*) versus spread lips (*right*).

Common Challenges

As with the /t/, finding the right spot for the PoA is a common challenge. However, because we are adding a pitch just before the burst, it does not have the same force as in the /t/ with only air pressure. Thus, the intraoral pressure is changing the tongue shape. You can also see the difference between the two in the tongue shapes (Figure 10–7).

In the /d/, the tongue root is not as elongated as it is in the /t/. In the latter, the air pressure shapes the tongue root more (elongation and a little dent in the bottom). The interaction between this mechanical compliance of the surface in the vicinity of the constriction and the tongue groove will help funnel the airstream with all its energy to the center of the teeth and not spread it to the side, losing the power. In the /d/ the noise component is much less and therefor doesn't require so much pressure build up. Hence, the difference in with more 'gentler' dents along the tongue and less elongation.

And yes, you probably guessed it, there is the prevoiced part that we ought to look out for. Because of the different PoA, it is often substituted with an /n/ (as in <u>n</u>oo<u>n</u>) instead of the very short voicing preceding the stop release. Again, using the hands to close your nose and possibly a spectrograph for monitoring will help with sensitizing the difference.

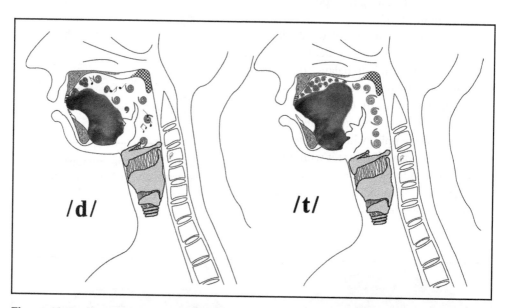

Figure 10–7. Juxtaposition of /d/ (*left*) and /t/ (*right*).

/g/ as in Gig

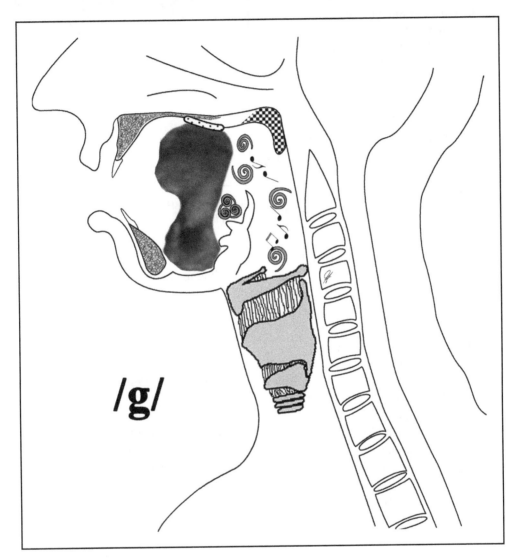

Figure 10–8. Ultrasound representation of /g/.

Articulatory Considerations

1. Physiological description
   a. The lips are apart and neutral.
   b. The tongue body is raised to create a seal across the soft palate, back molars, and the back (posterior) gum ridge.
   c. The velopharyngeal port is closed.
   d. The vocal folds come together (adducted), hence creating sound (pitch) only for a moment in prevoicing.

e. The air pressure is building up behind the tongue and soft palate seal.

f. Once the tongue releases the contact, the sound of the following vowel is released, and the turbulence creates the noise associated with the phoneme.

2. Step-by-step instructions

Remember the challenge in the consonants /k/ of an open, relaxed mouth while sealing the airflow through the tongue? Well, the same applies here and, as with /b/ and /d/, we also have to add a sound to it. But one step at a time.

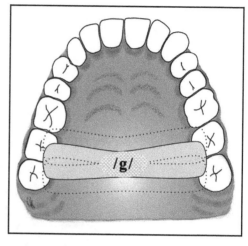

Figure 10–9. Possible places of articulation (PoA) for /g/.

- With your mouth still closed, find contact with the tongue surface (blade) on your hard palate. Also, feel how the sides of your tongue touch the molars and hence seal the entire mouth.
- Put your fingers on the joint that connects the jaw to your skull (temporomandibular joint [TMJ]). You can find that hinge in front of each ear (Chapter 2, Figure 2–4).
- Without pushing it, drop the jaw as far as you can in a relaxed manner, and with your fingers, feel how the bone (condyle) moves forward and bulges. Your larynx will also relax downward.

Now place your attention on your tongue.

- Allow the back of the tongue to relax (downward), elongating its trunk (see ultrasound image).
- Move the blade along the hard palate and find the spot (PoA) that makes the relaxation/drop of the trunk/back of the tongue and jaw easier (Figure 10–9). Should you have trouble moving the tongue along the palate, maybe you are curling the tip to guide your tongue. See the Common Challenges sections for help.
- Feel the contact of the tongue surface to the hard palate, imagine letting go of any tension in the trunk of the tongue, and allow it to elongate (see ultrasound image).
- If you are still feeling a lot of tension, reset. But before you start again, bite on the edges of your tongue and once you set the PoA again, imagine letting go of those edges.
- Once you are set again, phonate (on pitch) with a good pressure buildup to the point when it comes to a natural stop and release it without losing the sound and energy by collapsing your rib cage and/or closing the jaw. Imagine the direction of the release going back down into your throat instead of outward. That will help you to balance out the sudden pressure changes and turbulence without trying to push the air outward by engaging your larynx.

Common Challenges

Similar to the /k/ in Chapter 9, the challenge in this consonant is finding the right PoA. In speech without consonant resonance (CR), we only move the back/root of the tongue upward to establish contact with the palate. However, with the relaxed, dropped jaw, we are increasing the oral distance; hence, the root of the tongue needs to elongate and is therefore no longer the articulator that establishes contact with the PoA. Also, remember to find your vertically most comfortable PoA. As indicated in Figure 10–6, this can be in the vicinity of the transition of hard to soft palate and, most likely, will move a bit backward once you open the mouth. Furthermore, the release and elongation of the genioglossus, hyoglossus, palatoglossus (see the images in the preamble to Part II) as well as the side of the tongue edges are necessary to relieve this effort. For the latter, it helps to bite on the edges of your tongue, putting the focus and feeling on them, so you can imagine letting them go (retract). Also, remember the tongue depressor exercise in Chapter 4? Putting the depressor on the tip of the tongue will help you with the retraction and prevent the tip from curling and subsequently frees up the root of the tongue. A few repetitions of this exercise will help free up the tongue, and then you can start again to find your ideal PoA for the /g/.

Although we do not have a lot of "noise" within the consonant, the tension in the larynx may still occur for the very brief phonation. Remember the "let physics work for you" mantra. The release of the tongue contact to the palate is creating the characteristic noise associated with this consonant. Hence, there is no need to add any more muscular action by pushing harder, particularly not from the throat. In addition, the prevoicing should not be substituted with an /ŋ/ (as in si<u>ng</u>). Picturing the force of the release going backward into the mouth prevents the pushed tension in the larynx. Again, using the hands to close your nose and possibly a spectrograph for monitoring will help with sensitizing the difference.

11 Mid/Back Fricatives and the Aspirate— /h/ /χ/ /ç/ /ð/ /θ/

General Considerations

You are now probably going to ask why we are including two consonants, /ç/ and /χ/, that one does not even find in American English? This book is for both actors and singers, and in singing, we encounter them in other languages including German, Russian, Hebrew, Welsh, Irish, and Dutch. However, actors may also need them when they have to say something in one of those languages and/or when they need some percussive noise to express an emotional state. I am particularly thinking of fear-based screams that you do not want to solely create in your voice box (vocal folds) because that would harm your voice and most likely make you voiceless by the end of a performance. So, what can you do to avoid that? A scream has two main ingredients: high pitch and noise. The latter you can add through the phoneme /χ/. Following, you can see that the place of articulation (PoA) is at the soft palate and articulated with the back body of the tongue creating contact at the velum. This constriction creates a narrow pathway, causing turbulence, which is why we call the manner of articulation (MoA) a fricative. Combining high pitch with it gives you exactly what we hear in a scream. Of course, there is a bit more to

it (support through the body, etc.). Actors who want to become skilled in these kinds of specialties should explore the work of the theatrical voice trainer, Kate DeVore.

For singers, it is mainly a language that will require them to know how to pronounce these consonants. However, there is also a big controversy among the singing community regarding the /ç/ (as in "ich") in German that I would like to address here. This consonant does not exist in the English language which makes it even harder to master properly. From a physiological and acoustic standpoint, the different tongue shapes in the ultrasound images are obvious, and a look at the spectrogram clearly shows the difference between the two phonemes (Figure 11–1).

As you will see, the PoA is similar to that of /k/ (as in can). The difference, though, is that the airflow is not coming to a complete stop but still has a groove opening in the middle (medial) of the tongue. Thus, the constriction is creating the turbulence required for the noise. This is not an easy process to master, which is why a lot of times singers tend to substitute the /ç/ with a /ʃ/ (as in shine) or even a /k/ (as in can) which in comparison are easier to execute.

In addition to the challenge of the execution, in German classical singing (and Lieder, in particular), there are many who

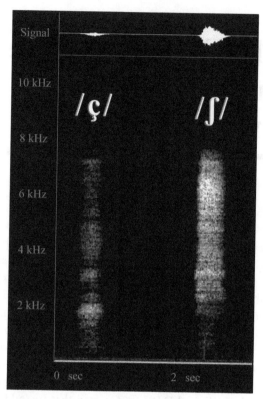

Figure 11–1. Comparison of /ç/ (*left*) and /ʃ/ (*right*).

argue that this is the proper phonation found in Germany. Unfortunately, that is not true. This is why we have to inject a note of caution here regarding the difference between dialect and standard/high German (sometimes also referred to as *Bühnenaussprache* [stage language]) or any other language for that matter. There are regional German places (e.g., the Rhineland) that use /ʃ/ instead of /ç/, though again, this is a dialect and does not constitute standard German.

But what does "standard German" actually mean? Johann Wolfgang Goethe (1749–1832), the German writer and statesman, was a big advocate—primarily for actors—of implementing rules for the artistic use of the German language. Though it is also not a secret that he did not repudiate his own very

Hessian-influenced colloquial language (e.g., *"ach neige, du Scherzensreiche ... "* (/ɑχ nʌˈɡə, du ʃɚtsənsrˇʌˈçə/ from Faust), one can still sense it in the rhyme *neische/reische* (König, 1994). Nonetheless, Theodor Siebs, the German philologist, in his first edition of *Deutsche Bühnenaussprache* in 1898, was the first to publish a codified use of the spoken word. This codex was primarily aimed at actors and later was adapted for public speakers, teachers, and so on. This is why one has to keep in mind that Siebs was adamant in promoting over-articulation of anything and everything for the sake of intelligibility in the challenging acoustic conditions in contemporary theaters. Fast-forward, and today we have the *Duden, Großes Wörterbuch der deutschen Aussprache* (GWdA), and *Deutsches Aus-*

prachewörterbuch (DAWB) as the most important dictionaries for the pronunciation of German. These latter are the first to give concrete details about phonologically stylistic differentiation within the codification. However, the *Duden* remains the market leader.

Although we have those three leading pronunciation dictionaries of the standard German language, even there we find a number of differences. However, these are more concerned with diphthongs, assorted vowels, and as we see later in Chapter 14, the realizations of various r-allophones. What they agree on, though, is that it is not appropriate to substitute /ç/ with /ʃ/ in German. This is why we need to be careful when we teach others German, or any language for that matter, and question if we truly know the appropriate pronunciation. When teaching in our native language, we have to be careful not to pass on dialect influenced by our upbringing or past. Similarly, when we teach another language, we have to ask ourselves if the person who taught us the language did so with the same considerations.

Research and technology have not yielded any new techniques but continue to expand our knowledge and show the efficacy of certain technical approaches to help illuminate and eliminate theories as well as unhealthy vocal practices. The best tribute to teaching is to continue learning, which I believe also means to continue questioning one's own and other's knowledge, so it does not become vestigial through routine.

/h/ as in <u>H</u>umble

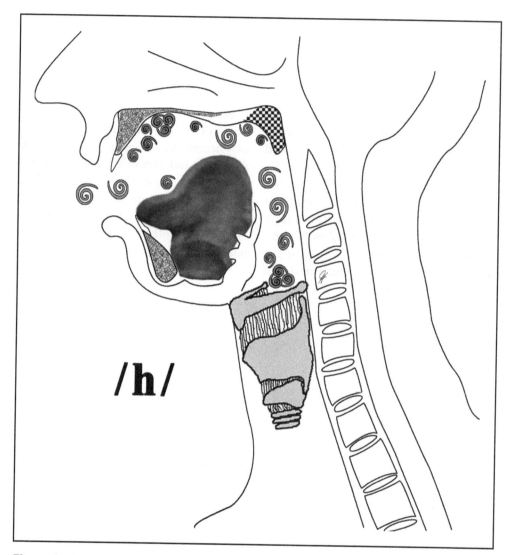

/h/

Figure 11–2. Ultrasound representation of /h/.

Articulatory Considerations

1. Physiological description
   a. The lips are apart and positioned for the following sound.
   b. The tongue is positioned for the following vowel.
   c. The velopharyngeal port is closed.
   d. The vocal folds are approximated (like a whisper).
   e. The turbulence is primarily created above the narrowest channel between tongue and palate and guided along the hard palate.

2. Step-by-step instructions

This may be one of the harder consonants to get acquainted with because there is almost no action required from the articulators. The /h/ could be compared to a whisper where the vocal folds are not vibrating and are only close enough to create a narrow passage that increases the airflow as it passes through, thus creating white noise.

- With your mouth still closed, put your fingers on the joint that connects the jaw to your skull (temporomandibular joint [TMJ]). You can find that hinge in front of each ear (see Chapter 2, Figure 2–4).
- Without pushing it, drop the jaw as far as you can in a relaxed manner and feel in your fingers how the bone (condyle) moves forward and bulges. Your larynx will also relax downward.
- Start to sustain a whisper on the vowel /ɑ/. It is like wanting to phonate (creating sound through a complete closure of the vocal folds) but holding off doing so just before it happens. Even if you cross into the phonation, notice how the airflow strokes the vocal folds before you make sound. Also, do you hear how it creates an audible white noise because of the turbulence created between the narrow gap?
- Try to reverse the direction in taking a deep breath while constricting the glottis (gap between the vocal folds). Do not worry, the increased force also increases the chances of unintentionally adding sound. The main thing is to raise your awareness of the air between the vocal folds.

Note: hearing white noise when taking a breath is a sign of tension within the larynx and should be addressed.

Now focus your attention on your tongue:

- With the newly gained awareness, go back to sustaining a whisper on the vowel /ɑ/ and change the tongue from a groove to no groove (see Chapter 4, Figure 4–11) or move it around. Notice how you change the spectrum (you will hear different phonemes) of the white noise? Some tongue shapes will have more intensity than others. Yes, the filter described in Chapters 5 and 7 is in action, changing the formants, meaning you can hear various vowels when changing the tongue. As with the plosives, imagine the direction of the air going back down into your lungs instead of outward. That will help you maintain an equilibrium of your approximated vocal folds without pushing it outward by engaging your larynx or even collapsing your rib cage.

Common Challenges

As you could see from the step-by-step instructions, the /h/ does not take on a particular articulatory description on its own, which is why some may refer to it as a voiceless vowel. Similar to other voiceless consonants, it is not uncommon to find muscle tension in the larynx in order to ensure audibility of the consonant. Because the whisper lacks in intensity and cannot be heard very well or from far away, maximum consonant resonance (CR) is crucial and can be accomplished by bringing the vocal folds close enough together so they start to vibrate just a little: this is called a stage whisper (a mixture of a lot of whisper and a little bit of a pitch). However, as with all voiceless consonants, we are working within the laws of physics to help make air audible by narrowing the pathway through constriction within the vocal tract. In this case, we rely solely on the vocal folds and a narrowing of the tract above the glottis. All of this should not be accomplished through tension within the larynx. Additionally, dependent on the demand, the tongue shape can help create either more friction, hence higher frequencies within the vocal tract (e.g., /i/), or amplification of the turbulence within the glottis (e.g., /ɑ/).

Note: Knowing how to consciously add breath to one's voice can be quite useful for stylistic reasons. Adding an intentional gap between the vocal folds to let some air leak out will give the voice a husky quality. A novice singer, however, may be straining so hard to accomplish a breathy voice that she ends up tensing multiple muscles in the larynx and inadvertently holds the vocal folds apart. Of course, the same is true for a singer or speaker (like muscle tension disorder [MTD]) that has an airy or breathy voice as a baseline. Working on breath support and laryngeal relaxation may be advisable.

/χ/ as in Ug<u>h</u>! (as in "A<u>ch</u>!" in German)

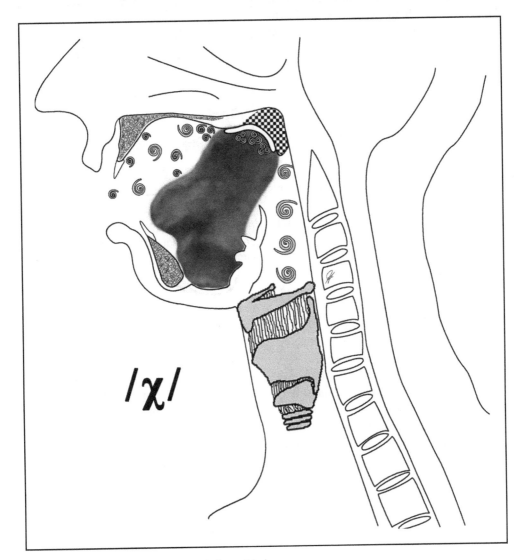

Figure 11–3. Ultrasound representation of /χ/.

Articulatory Considerations

1. Physiological description
   a. The lips are apart and neutral.
   b. The tongue body is raised to create contact with the uvula.
   c. The velopharyngeal port is closed.
   d. The vocal folds are not together (abducted), hence no sound.
   e. Air goes through the constricting narrow channel of the tongue and uvula (PoA) causing turbulence that creates the noise associated with the phoneme.

2. Step-by-step instructions

As mentioned at the beginning of this chapter, this consonant cannot be found in American English. But as singers, one has to sing in many other languages, and as actors/actresses, one has to mimic the sound for various reasons (e.g., dialect, scream, etc.).

- With the mouth still closed, put your fingers on the joint that connects the jaw to your skull (TMJ). You can find that hinge in front of each ear (Chapter 2, Figure 2–4).
- Without pushing it, drop the jaw as far as you can in a relaxed manner and feel in your fingers how the bone (condyle) moves forward and bulges. Your larynx will also relax downward.

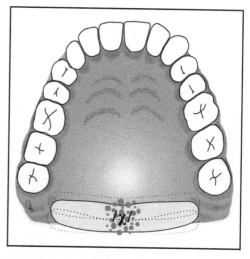

Figure 11–4. Possible places of articulation (PoA) for /χ/. Turbulence and flapping in the center of the tongue are indicated by gray/blue circles.

Now focus your attention on your tongue.

- Allow the root of the tongue to relax (downward) as well, so it can elongate its trunk (see ultrasound image).
- Move the body of the tongue along the hard palate as far back to the soft palate/velum and find the spot (PoA) that makes the relaxation/drop of the trunk/back of the tongue and jaw easier (Figure 11–4).
- Feel the contact of the tongue surface to the velum and imagine releasing any tension underneath in the trunk of the tongue to allow it to elongate (see ultrasound image). Also, keep the tip of the tongue low and prevent it from curling up, which would prevent the rest of the tongue body from forming. A tongue depressor may be helpful (see Common Challenges later).
- If you are still feeling a lot of tension, reset. But before you start again, bite on the edges of your tongue, and once you set the PoA again, imagine releasing those edges.

- Once you are set again, prepare for a good airflow and energize the /χ/. Ideally, you should hear a lot of white noise mixed with some low pulsating, almost like a trill, noise. The latter is the uvula flapping against the tongue surface; it may need some time to actually start doing so. It is somewhat like a reversed snore, only now the airstream is passing between uvula and tongue rather than the uvula, tongue, and sinuses. In order to get a feel for it, you may want to experiment this somewhat noisy exercise: try to sniff back, as if you want to clear your nose from congested mucus or simulate a snore, and feel the flapping uvula. This will give you a sense of where the uvula is and what the turbulence between the constriction of the contact area feels like. Once you establish the sensation, try to replicate the same flapping for the consonant /χ/. As always, do not push it too hard, and imagine the direction going backward rather than outward.

Common Challenges

When you look at the ultrasound image, the muscle of the uvula closes the nasopharynx with its back part (anteriorly). The rest of the connective tissue is still relaxed and will act like a noisy flatter valve, though it can be challenging to keep this balance between tension and relaxation (see Chapter 2 "tensegrity") and may, as a result, lead to tension only.

The process starts with the tongue. To move the front (anterior) body of the tongue toward the uvula, both the root and the tip of the tongue have to move accordingly, elongating the root of the tongue and relaxing or, dependent on the tongue length, possibly retracting the tip (apex) of the tongue. It is not uncommon to see the tip starting the movement of the tongue body by curling backward, creating tension with the tongue and, due to the collective pushback, subsequently the uvula. As discussed in Chapter 4, a tongue depressor or something similar can help keep the tip under control and ease the tension within the tongue and genioglossus, respectively.

The uvula is a conic projection from the back (posterior) edge of the middle of the soft palate. The consonant /χ/ is not a stop consonant (the airflow comes to a complete hold before the release) but rather a constriction of airflow through a narrow channel. In the side (sagittal) view of the ultrasound, it looks as if the tongue completely seals the airway at the PoA. However, it is only the sides of the tongue that somewhat seal the area, whereas in the middle, we actually have a little groove that creates the narrow channel between tongue and uvula (see Figure 11–4). Thus, we have to make sure to direct the airstream along the center of the tongue, rather than to the sides.

This is where our "let physics work for you" comes into play. The flapping occurs because of the aerodynamic conditions: the back of the tongue is placed close enough to the uvula (a soft part), and an air jet of sufficient strength starts a repeating pattern of closing and opening. Thus, there is no need to add any musculature action such as pushing, particularly not from the throat. Imagining the airflow going backward into the mouth will help prevent the upward push in the larynx and keep the balance of the constriction between tongue and uvula. Additionally, keep the rib cage expanded/lifted through the support with your lower abdominal muscles and maintain a relaxed, dropped jaw.

/ç/ as in I<u>ch</u> (German) or <u>H</u>ue (English)

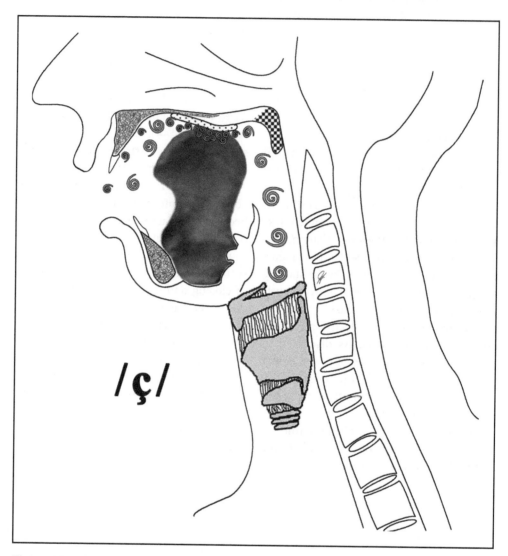

Figure 11–5. Ultrasound representation of /ç/.

Articulatory Considerations

1. Physiological description
   a. The lips are apart and neutral.
   b. The tongue body is raised to create contact with the transition of hard and soft palate.
   c. The velopharyngeal port is closed.
   d. The vocal folds are not together (abducted), hence no sound.
   e. Air goes through the constricting narrow channel of the tongue and palate (PoA), causing turbulence

that creates the noise associated with the phoneme.

2. Step-by-step instructions

As mentioned at the beginning of this chapter, this is one of the most controversial consonants that is often erroneously substituted with /ʃ/. But as you will see, there are no similarities in either the MoA or the PoA.

▨ With your mouth closed, breathe through your nose and feel where your tongue is. In this position, the entire tongue should be resting on the roof of your mouth (feel the tongue surface making contact with the palate), providing an internal support system for the upper jaw.

▨ Now try to create a groove by releasing in the middle of the tongue while maintaining contact with the edges (Figure 11–6). Imagine the genioglossus (GG) depressing downward. It helps to put the top of two fingers underneath the chin to feel the push from the GG against the fingers (see also Chapter 4).

▨ With the little tunnel running through the middle of the tongue, open the

mouth a little and start to breathe through it and feel the cold air stroking along the surface. Because of the narrow nature of that tunnel, you should also hear the air rubbing against the surfaces, creating a hissing sound. Due to the arch in the front of the palate, the hissing is stronger on the exhalation.

Add the low mandible maneuver (LMM):

▨ Put your fingers on the joint that connects the jaw to your skull (TMJ). You can find that hinge in front of each ear (see Chapter 2, Figure 2–4).

▨ Without pushing it, drop the jaw in a relaxed manner as far as you can and feel in your fingers how the bone (condyle) moves forward and bulges. Your larynx will also relax downward.

▨ Allow the back of the tongue to relax, downward as well, so it can elongate its trunk (see ultrasound image).

▨ Similar to the consonants /k/, the PoA may move back a little along the hard palate once you relax/drop the trunk/back of the tongue and jaw (Figure 11–7).

▨ Feel the contact of the tongue edges to the hard palate and imagine letting any tension in the trunk (root) of the tongue and allow it to elongate (see ultrasound image).

▨ With good support from your lower abdominal muscles, energize the /ç/ and notice again the turbulence along the tunnel in the middle of your tongue.

Common Challenges

If we do not recognize a foreign sound, it is natural to mimic or use the most approximate sound in our own language to replace

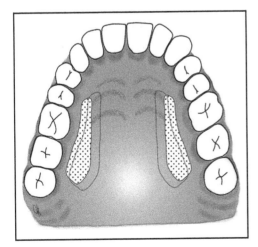

Figure 11–6. Place of articulation (PoA) for /ç/.

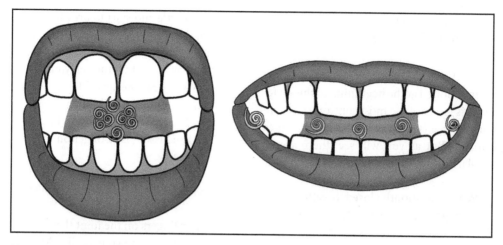

Figure 11–7. Spreading of the lips (*left*) versus relaxed, slightly protruded lips (*right*) for /ç/.

it. However, in English, the closest sound may be an overexaggerated /h/, as in <u>h</u>uge, and not /ʃ/, as in <u>sh</u>ow. As we have seen in the stop consonant /k/ (as in <u>c</u>an), maintaining contact to the hard palate while elongating the rest of the tongue underneath may be the most challenging part in this consonant. This is often a good way to think of it: the surface of the tongue edges touch the palate, and everything underneath relaxes. Or look at the graphics in the preamble to Part II and imagine the release and elongation of the genioglossus, hyoglossus, palatoglossus, as well as the side of the tongue edges. For the latter, it helps to bite on the edges of your tongue, placing your focus and feeling on

them, so you can imagine letting them go (retracting) instead of spreading them.

Of course, unlike in the /k/, the edges of the tongue are functioning as the PoA, funneling the air along the center of the tongue. On the spectrogram (Figure 11–8), you can see the effect of the change of our two chambers (front/oral and back/pharyngeal, discussed in Chapters 5 and 7) quite clearly: the various bright spots (formants; Chapter 7) are more distinctly noticeable than on the right; higher as well as lower frequencies are noticeable on the left where CR and the lower mandible maneuver (LMM) are applied; and an increase in measured amplitude (signal).

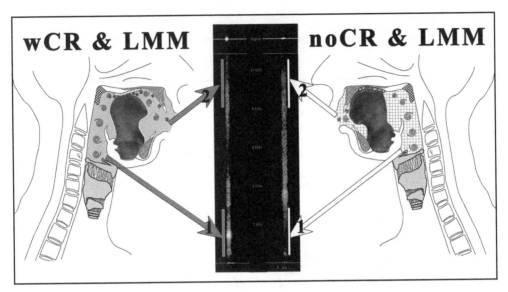

Figure 11–8. Spectrogram of the consonant /ç/ executed with consonant resonant (CR) and lower mandible maneuver (LMM) (*left, gray/red*) and without (*right, tiles/green*).

/ð/ as in <u>Th</u>at

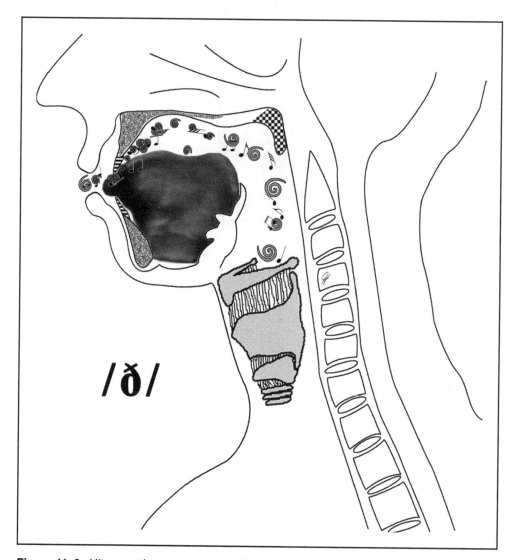

Figure 11–9. Ultrasound representation of /ð/.

Articulatory Considerations

1. Physiological description
   a. The lips are apart though a little protruded (like a tube).
   b. The mandible is lowered slightly in back (LMM, second strategy).
   c. The tongue tip is shifted forward and rests in between the teeth.
   d. The velopharyngeal port is closed.
   e. The vocal folds come together (adducted), hence creating sound.
   f. Airflow is through the constriction formed by the teeth and tongue

front, causing turbulence that creates the noise accompanying the phoneme's sound.

2. Step-by-step instructions

Although a very frequent consovowel (pitch + noise; Chapter 7) in English, it can cause considerable difficulties for both native and non-native speakers of American English.

■ Put the tip of the tongue between your teeth and hold it with a gentle squeeze (PoA). Both upper and lower teeth should have contact with your tongue.
■ Put your fingers on the joint that connects the jaw to your skull (TMJ). You can find that hinge in front of each ear (see Chapter 2, Figure 2–4).
■ With the tongue tip between the teeth, drop the back of the jaw (posterior mandible) in a relaxed manner and feel in your fingers how the bone (condyle) moves forward and bulges. Your larynx will also relax downward (LMM, second strategy, Chapter 3), creating room in the pharynx.
■ Start to sustain on a pitch and feel both the vibration (which are the reflections of the sound within the oral cavity) in your teeth and on your tongue surface as well as the friction of the turbulence from the constriction teeth and tongue.
■ Make sure the back of the tongue is relaxed and not trying to push toward the action in the front. And, "let physics work for you" (feel the pressure and airflow going backward, preventing the larynx and tongue from tensing up).

Common Challenges

You may be surprised, but sustaining such a "noisy" pitch can often be a challenge. The

airstream is channeled centrally through the front of the tongue and teeth, which can be quite ticklish and very loud at first. Both may evoke a subconscious reaction to not squeeze the tongue enough, so the noise does not "disturb" the sound. I often say, "don't make the /ð/ too pretty by only phonating the pitch; the noise is part of the consovowel's identity." Let us try it out. Sustain a pitch where the teeth barely touch the tongue. Do you hear a lot of noise? Do you feel the air spreading to the sides, losing the energy? Does it tickle less? And now the reverse, sustain the pitch while squeezing and pushing really hard. Did the airflow and sound stop? We need the balance of the two to produce this voiced interdental fricative.

Although due to the combination of sound and noise this consovowel is not made with as much force as its voiceless counterpart /θ/ (as in wi<u>th</u>), the spreading of the lips as an instinctual counteraction to increase the airflow can still be found. The lip rounding in combination with some tongue guidance (groove, elongation) will help funnel the airstream with all its energy to the center of the teeth and not spread it to the side, losing the power. It helps to put your index fingers in the corner of the lips to help counteract the spreading.

Concomitant with that, more often than not, tension in the larynx emanates in order to "create" the noise part of the consovowel. This is where our "let physics work for you" comes into play. The tongue tip between the teeth forms a constriction that in turn creates friction, which is the noise part associated with the consonant. Hence, there is no need to separately add any musculature action by pushing harder, particularly not from the throat. Imagining the airflow going backward into the mouth will help prevent the upward push in the larynx and keep the balance of the constriction between tongue front and teeth.

Last, but not least, care must be taken to only place the tongue tip between the space of the front teeth and not sandwich the entire tongue along the side. Once the tongue reaches the canines, you may be pushing too hard and spreading both tongue and lips.

/θ/ as in <u>Th</u>in

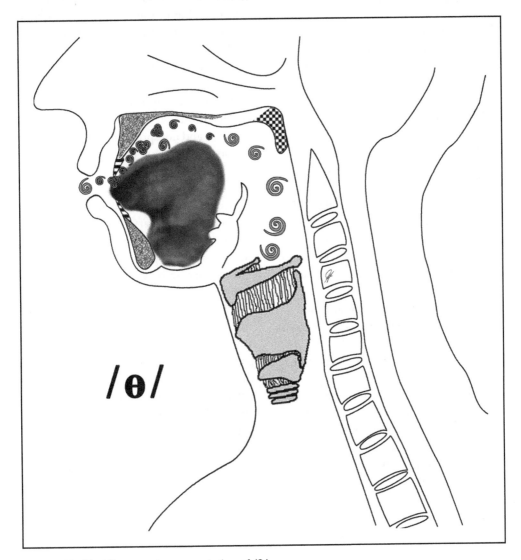

Figure 11–10. Ultrasound representation of /θ/.

Articulatory Considerations

1. Physiological description
   a. The lips are apart though a little protruded (like a tube)
   b. The mandible is lowered slightly in back (LMM, second strategy).
   c. The tongue tip is shifted forward and rests in between the teeth.
   d. The velopharyngeal port is closed.
   e. The vocal folds are not together (abducted), hence no sound.
   f. Airflow is through the constriction formed by the teeth and tongue

front, causing turbulence that creates the noise accompanying the phoneme's sound.

2. Step-by-step instruction

It is similar in the production to its voiced cognate except it is made with a little more force.

- Put the tip of the tongue between your teeth and hold it with a gentle squeeze (PoA). Both upper and lower teeth should have contact with your tongue.
- Put your fingers on the joint that connects the jaw to your skull (TMJ). You can find that hinge in front of each ear (see Chapter 2, Figure 2–4).
- With the tongue tip between the teeth, drop the back of the jaw (posterior mandible) in a relaxed manner and feel in your fingers how the bone (condyle) moves forward and bulges. Your larynx will also relax downward (LMM, second strategy, Chapter 3), creating room in the pharynx.
- Start to energize the consonants with a good lower abdominal supported airflow and feel the friction of the turbulence between tongue front and teeth. If the flow stops, you are squeezing and/or pushing too hard; if there is little or no resistance, it is too loose (little noise).
- Make sure the back of the tongue is relaxed/elongated. Imagine the airstream going backward, instead of trying to push it toward the action in the front, constricting the larynx and tongue.

Common Challenges

Although the articulatory considerations are straightforward and similar to its voiced counterpart /ð/, this consonant can be chal-

lenging, and not only for non-native speakers. The consonant production is solely composed of air and friction. This is why the spreading of the lips as an instinctual counteraction to the increase in airflow is likely to occur. The lip rounding in combination with some tongue guidance (groove, elongation; see the dimple in the ultrasound representation earlier) will help funnel the airstream with all its energy to the center of the teeth and not spread it to the side, losing the power. It helps to put your index fingers in the corner of the lips to counteract the spreading.

Concomitant with that, more often than not, tension in the larynx emanates in order to "create" the noise part of the consonant. As I always say, "let physics work for you." The tongue tip between the teeth forms a constriction that in turn creates friction, which is the noise part associated with the consonant. Hence, there is no need to add any musculature action by pushing harder, particularly not from the throat. Imagining the airflow to go backward into the mouth will help prevent the constriction in the larynx and keep the balance of the constriction between tongue front and teeth.

Last, but not least, we need to make sure that we place the tongue tip between the space of the front teeth and do not sandwich the entire tongue along the side. Once the tongue reaches the canines, you may be pushing too hard and spreading both tongue and lips.

References

Deutsches Aussprachewörterbuch (DAWB). (2009). Hrsg.: Krech, E.-M./Stock, E./Hirschfeld, U./ Anders, L.C. Berlin.

Duden. (2015). *Das Aussprachewörterbuch*. Bd. 6 (7th ed.), Komplett überarbeitete und aktualisierte Auflage. Berlin.

Großes Wörterbuch der deutschen Aussprache. (1982). Hrsg.: Krech, E.-M./Kurka, E./Stelzig, H./Stock, E./Stötzer, U./Teske, R. Leipzig: VEB Bibliographisches Institut.

König, W. (1994). *dtv-Atlas zur deutschen Sprach.* Tafeln und Texte. Mit Mundarten-Karte. (11th ed.). München.

Siebs, Th. (1898). *Deutsche Bühnenaussprache* (15th ed.). Berlin, Köln, Leipzig.

12 Front Fricatives—/s/ /ʃ/ /f/

General Considerations

As we have already seen, fricative sounds are produced by a narrow constriction at some point along the length of the vocal tract, created by placing two articulators close together. This creates a turbulent airstream that in turn generates the noise (friction) associated with the consonant. In other words, because the high velocity of the air jet formed by that narrow constriction hits an obstruction, such as the teeth. In comparison, the precision of the place of articulation (PoA) of the fricative has to be greater than in the nasal or stop consonants. Why?

In a stop or nasal consonant, you hold one articulator against another (e.g., /n/, as in noon), tongue tip against the gum ridge above your upper teeth (alveolar ridge). From a motor sensory perspective, this makes it a bit easier to set up and shape the consonant. In a fricative, we have to (a) maintain a precisely shaped channel for a turbulent airstream to be produced and (b) hold that exactly defined shape for a noticeable period of time. Any change in the formation of the filter changes the acoustic end result. Thus, we need to watch out even more on how the rest of the tongue is shaped in relation to the other articulators.

In general, the resonant frequency in the fricatives spans from high to low, moving with the PoA front to back. It all depends on the volume of the cavity between the PoA and the lips. The spectral energy in front fricatives (dental, alveolar ridge) has higher frequencies (approximately above 4 kHz), while that of palatal fricatives naturally lies lower at approximately above 2.5 kHz (Howard & Murphy, 2008). This is why, as artists on stage, we need to remember our two-chamber hallway metaphor (Chapter 5) to have maximum consonant resonance (CR) because higher frequencies, for instance in /ʃ/ (as in shine), do not travel well in larger or acoustically poor halls. Thus, pharyngeal openness (throat) is crucial to add lower frequencies and avoid anti-resonances (Chapter 7).

/s/ as in <u>S</u>un

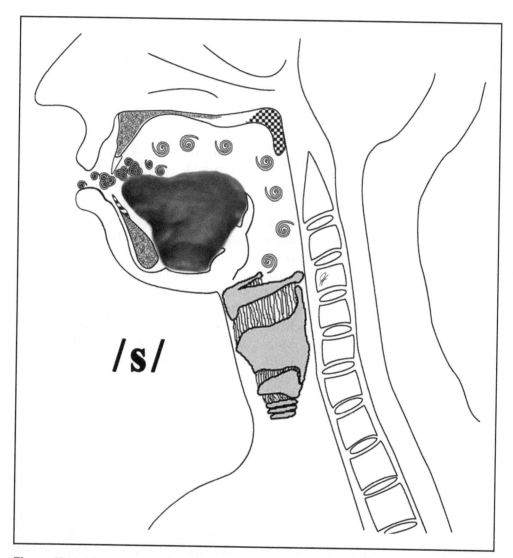

Figure 12–1. Ultrasound representation of /s/.

Articulatory Considerations

1. Physiological description
   a. The lips are slightly apart though a little rounded (like a tube).
   b. The jaw (mandible) is lowered in the back (low mandible maneuver [LMM], second strategy).
   c. The tongue tip may be at the lower front teeth or a little raised. The blade and body of the tongue are depressed, creating a groove along the midline; the tongue edges make contact with the upper gum ridge.
   d. The velopharyngeal port is closed.

e. The vocal folds are not together (abducted), hence no sound.

f. The airstream is channeled through the groove in the tongue and breaks against the upper gum ridge (alveolar ridge) and front teeth, creating turbulence.

2. Step-by-step instructions

The /s/ consonant may seem simple and may be the most frequently occurring fricative in the English language (Edwards, 2003). It is also among the most difficult; speech-language pathologists spend countless hours correcting this speech sound error. Non-native speakers of American English do not usually have a problem with it.

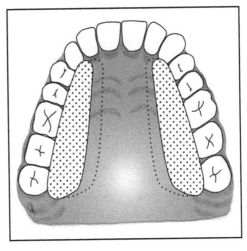

Figure 12–2. Contact of tongue edges with the upper gum ridge for /s/.

- Round your lips and put the tip of the tongue (apex) to the lower front teeth.
- Put your fingers on the joint that connects the jaw to your skull (temporomandibular joint [TMJ]). You can find that hinge in front of each ear (see Chapter 2, Figure 2–4).
- Drop the back of the jaw (posterior mandible) in a relaxed manner, and feel in your fingers how the bone (condyle) moves forward and bulges. Your larynx will also relax downward (LMM, second strategy, Chapter 3), creating room in the back of the mouth (pharynx).
- Depress the front blade of the tongue to a groove, imaging a depression of the genioglossus (see the images in the preamble to Part II) as if you were holding a little bolus of water. With the groove, the tongue tip will retract, moving a little away from the lower teeth. For more help on the groove, refer to Chapter 4.
- Once you create the groove, you will feel the edges on the upper gum ridge more prominently from back to front (Figure 12–2). Should you not feel them

in the front or at all, you may have dropped the jaw too far.

- Take a breath and feel the cold air in that little groove and around the edges of your teeth.
- Now energize the /s/, channeling the airstream along the center groove line of your tongue against the upper teeth. Notice the turbulence in that narrow constriction.
- Make sure the back of the tongue is relaxed and not trying to push toward the action in the front. And, "let physics work for you" (feel the pressure and airflow going backward, preventing the larynx and tongue from tensing up).

Common Challenges

As with other consonants that we already visited, because of the voiceless nature, the /s/ requires some force. Hence, spreading of the lips as an instinctual counteraction to increase the airflow can always occur (Figure 12–3). The lip rounding in combination with the tongue guidance (groove) will help funnel the airstream with all its energy to

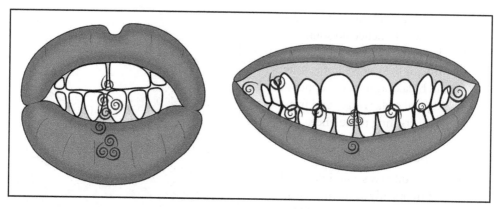

Figure 12–3. Relaxed, round lips (*left*) versus spread lips (*right*) for /s/.

the center of the teeth and not spread it to the side, losing power and lower frequencies. It helps to put your index fingers in the corner of the lips to help counteract the spreading.

The LMM can be another obstacle. Not lowering and relaxing the jaw (mandible) and concomitantly the back of the tongue will reduce the space in the back of the mouth (pharynx) and push the tongue mass forward (making the space in the front even narrower and without groove). As a result, the lower frequencies are being canceled out (pharyngeal constriction), and the higher frequencies are scattered and weak (missing groove).

Last, let us discuss the tongue tip (apex). As mentioned at the beginning of this chapter, in fricatives we do not push the tongue tip (apex) against the upper gum ridge (alveolar) or teeth for that matter. We have to maintain a precise shape of the tongue, particularly the tip, in close proximity of the lower teeth. It is possible that efforts to either make the groove or maintain the position and shape may be initiated by the tongue tip, making it curl too much. This takes away the higher frequencies and, as you see in our next consonant, modifies the phoneme from /s/ to a more /ʃ/-like (<u>sh</u>ine) phoneme.

/ʃ/ as in Shine

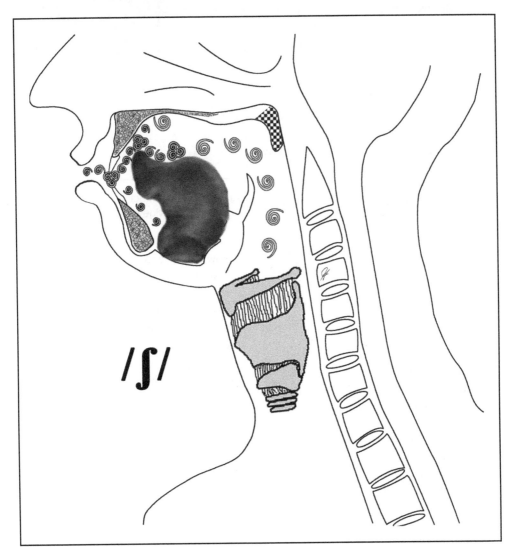

/ʃ/

Figure 12–4. Ultrasound representation of /ʃ/.

Articulatory Considerations

1. Physiological description
   a. The lips are slightly apart, rounded, and protruded.
   b. The jaw (mandible) is lowered in the back (LMM, second strategy).
   c. The tongue tip (apex) is curled. The blade and body of the tongue are depressed, creating a groove along the midline; the tongue edges make contact with the upper gum ridge.
   d. The velopharyngeal port is closed.

e. The vocal folds are not together (abducted), hence no sound.

f. The airstream is channeled through the groove in the tongue and breaks against the gum ridge, palate, and front teeth, creating turbulence.

2. Step-by-step instructions

The /ʃ/ is one of the most acoustically powerful fricatives. It may have similarities with the /s/, though as the ultrasound clearly shows, it does have a distinct difference.

■ Round your lips and put the tip of the tongue (apex) to the lower front teeth.

■ Put your fingers on the joint that connects the jaw to your skull (TMJ). You can find that hinge in front of each ear (see Chapter 2, Figure 2–4).

■ Drop the back of the jaw (posterior mandible) in a relaxed manner and feel in your fingers how the bone (condyle) moves forward and bulges. Your larynx will also relax downward (LMM, second strategy, Chapter 3), creating room in the back of the mouth (pharynx).

■ Depress the front blade of the tongue to a groove, imagining a depression of the genioglossus (see images in the preamble to Part II) as if holding a little bolus of water. With the groove, retract and curl the tongue tip upward, toward the gum ridge (alveolar). For more help on the groove, refer to Chapter 4.

■ Once you create the groove, you will feel the edges on the upper gum ridge more prominently from back to front (Figure 12–5). Should you not feel them in the front or at all, you may have dropped the jaw too far.

■ Take a breath and feel the cold air stroking the tip of the tongue and around the edges of your teeth.

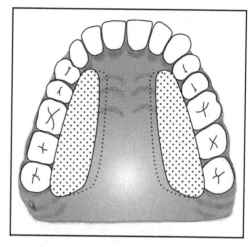

Figure 12–5. Contact of tongue edges with the upper gum ridge for /ʃ/.

■ Now energize the /ʃ/, channeling the airstream along the center groove line of your tongue, against the upper palate and teeth. Notice the turbulence in that narrow constriction.

■ Make sure the back of the tongue is relaxed and not trying to push toward the action in the front. And, "let physics work for you" (feel the pressure and airflow going backward, preventing the larynx and tongue from tensing up).

Common Challenges

First, it should be noted that /ʃ/ can be made in two ways, with the tip of the tongue up or down. However, on stage we are always trying to find the maximum CR in order to maintain the overall resonance and secure intelligibility. This is why we are using the curled tip of the tongue as well as the rounded lips. Acoustically, it lowers the frequency (lengthening of the vocal tract by added lip rounding and lower velocity) while maintaining the higher frequencies for the consonants' identity (remember the two-chamber hallway metaphor).

Sometimes, the curling of the tongue tip or keeping it in close proximity to the palate can be challenging. To make it easier, I suggest you first make contact with the palate (sealing it like a stop consonant), heightening the awareness of the position of the tongue tip. Next, build up the pressure behind it and feel the increase in the mouth (oral cavity), particularly on the surface of the tongue (like expanding the groove). Also, be sure to keep everything centered and do not push sideways. Then release the tip from the palate, opening just a little bit, and notice the "hizzing" sound (higher frequencies) created by the air jet passing through the narrow constriction, breaking against the gum ridge and teeth. Basically, we just made a /tʃ/ (as in ca<u>tch</u>), which is phonating /t/ and /ʃ/ in close succession. Toggle back and forth between the two and notice the little movement necessary for the tip of the tongue to release and—our primary interest—its close proximity to the palate. Once you are comfortable with the movement, leave the /t/ out and sustain only on the /ʃ/. Of course, with all the attention focused on the front of the mouth, the jaw and back of the tongue may have become stiff and will need to relax again (see step-by-step instructions presented earlier).

As with /s/, a spreading of the lips as an instinctive counteraction to increase the airflow can always occur (see Figure 12–3). The lip rounding in combination with the tongue guidance (groove) will help funnel the airstream with all its energy to the center of the teeth and not spread it to the side, losing power and lower frequencies. It helps to put your index fingers in the corner of the lips to help counteract the spreading.

The LMM can be another obstacle. Not lowering and relaxing the jaw (mandible) and, simultaneously, the back of the tongue will reduce the space in the pharynx and push the tongue mass forward (making the space in the front even narrower and without a groove). As a result, the lower frequencies are canceled out (pharyngeal constriction), and the higher frequencies are scattered and weak (missing groove).

/f/ as in <u>F</u>ine

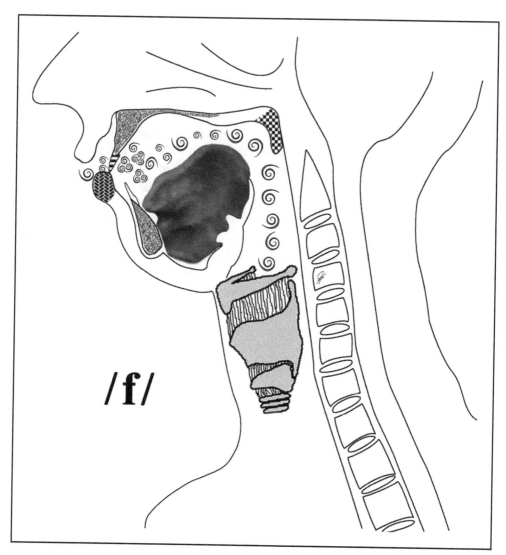

/f/

Figure 12–6. Ultrasound representation of /f/.

Articulatory Considerations

1. Physiological description
   a. The jaw (mandible) is lowered in the back (LMM, second strategy).

   b. The inner border of the lower lip is slightly rounded and raised to contact the upper teeth.
   c. The tongue tip (apex) may touch the lower jaw ridge on the bottom of the mouth behind the lower

teeth. The blade and body of the tongue are depressed, creating a groove along the midline.

  d. The velopharyngeal port is closed.

  e. The vocal folds are not together (abducted), hence no sound.

  f. The airstream is channeled along the groove through the light closure of the lower lip and upper teeth, thus creating friction.

2. Step-by-step instructions

The outgoing airflow creates a friction noise because of the constriction lip-teeth (labio-dental) obstruction. But as always, we have to start with building the resonance around it.

▨ Put your fingers on the joint that connects the jaw to your skull (TMJ). You can find that hinge in front of each ear (see Chapter 2, Figure 2–4).

▨ Drop the back of the jaw (posterior mandible) in a relaxed manner and feel in your fingers how the bone (condyle) moves forward and bulges. Your larynx will also relax downward (LMM, second strategy, Chapter 3), creating room in the pharynx.

▨ Set the vowel /ɑ/, depress the front blade of the tongue to a groove; imagine a depression of the genioglossus (see images in Part II) as if you were holding a little scoop of ice cream without allowing it to touch your teeth. For more help on the groove, have a look at Chapter 4. The tongue tip may touch the lower jaw ridge on the bottom of the mouth behind the lower teeth. The back of the tongue elongates with the second strategy of the LMM.

▨ Take a breath and slightly protrude both upper and lower lips. Raise the slightly more rounded and protruded lower lip to make contact with its inner border and upper teeth.

▨ Energize the /f/, guiding the airstream along the center groove line of your tongue to the middle of the PoA. Notice the turbulence at that narrow constriction between the inner aspect of the lower lip and the upper teeth. Feel the back pressure, possibly on the tongue surface, because of the limited outlet.

Common Challenges

In general, the influence of the vowel environment can be greater on some consonants than on others. Furthermore, the friction-like noise created by the lip-teeth (labio-dental) obstruction makes the /f/ an acoustically weak sound, similar to the theta /θ/. In order to create maximum CR, the vowel /ɑ/ with the LMM (Chapter 3) has shown to be the most effective vowel.

The same as in our previous consonants, spreading of the lips as an instinctual counteraction to increase the airflow can always occur (Figure 12–7). The lip rounding in combination with the tongue guidance (groove) will help funnel the airstream with all its energy to the center of the teeth and not spread it to the side, losing power and lower frequencies. It helps to put your index fingers in the corner of the lips to help counteract the spreading. It will also help prevent the cheeks from puffing up, which would also be an indicator of losing the energy to the side.

Concomitant with that, more often than not, tension emanates in the larynx in order to "create" the noise part of the consonant. This is again a case of letting physics work for you. The contact of the upper incisors and the lower lip forms a constriction that in turn creates friction, which is the noise part associated with the consonant. Hence,

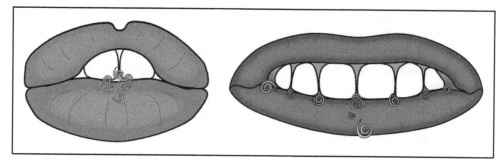

Figure 12–7. Relaxed, round lips (*left*) versus spread lips (*right*) for /f/.

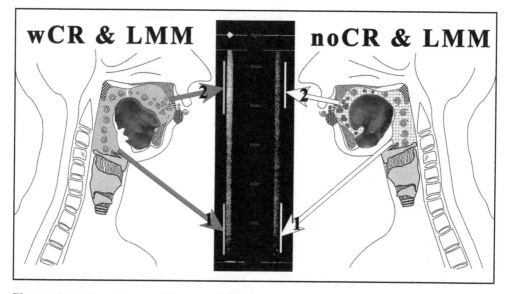

Figure 12–8. Spectrogram of the consonant /f/ executed with consonant resonance and lower mandible maneuver (*left, gray/red*) and without (*right, tiles/green*).

there is no need to separately add any musculature action by pushing harder, particularly not from the throat. Imagining the airflow going backward into the mouth will help prevent the upward push in the larynx and keep the balance of the constriction between lip and teeth.

Finally, look at the spectrogram (Figure 12–8). The size and shape of our two chambers again have significant impact on the acoustic end result of the /f/. Similar to that which we have seen before, the higher

and lower frequencies are affected, as well as the intensity (signal).

References

Edwards, H. T. (2003). *Applied phonetics: The sounds of American English* (3rd ed.). Clifton Park, NY: Thomson.

Howard, D. M., & Murphy, D. T. (2008). *Voice science, acoustics and recording.* San Diego, CA: Plural Publishing.

13 Front Voiced Fricatives—/z/ /ʒ/ /v/

General Considerations

In this chapter, we continue our fricatives, the phonemes in which a turbulent airstream is produced within the vocal tract. This also means that the same general consideration will apply. Except now the noise and turbulence are blended with a pitch; thus, we are talking about a consovowel (see Chapter 7). As simple as it may sound, this addition makes keeping the balance between the high intraoral pressure and the sound production quite challenging.

Why? This occurs because now the air jet has two "checkpoints," if you will: one at the vocal folds (glottis); and one at the teeth/lip. Both have to be supplied with efficient airflow. Similar to what we have seen for the stop and prevoiced consonants (see Chapters 9 and 10), the ultrasound images show similarities yet significant changes in their shape. It is again the difference in the interoral pressure. Thus, a passive displacement of the tongue surface and, as with voiceless fricatives, particularly, the tongue body/root occurs due to the increase in pressure (Figure 13–1).

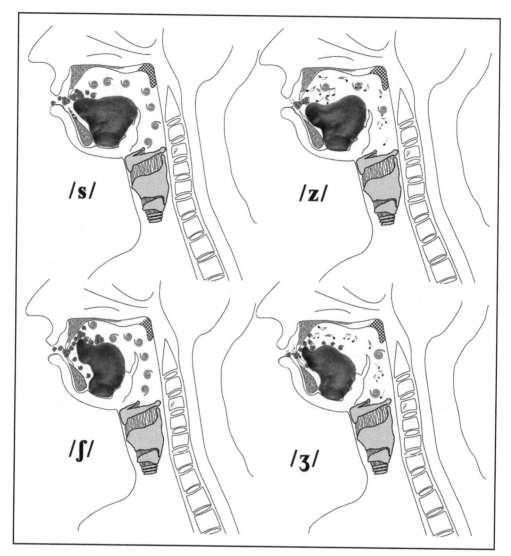

Figure 13–1. Juxtaposition of voiceless (*left*) and voiced (*right*) fricatives.

/z/ as in Zebra

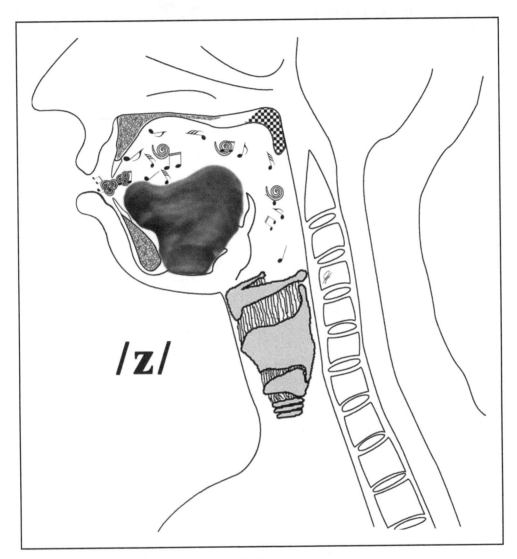

Figure 13–2. Ultrasound representation of /z/.

Articulatory Considerations

1. Physiological description
   a. The lips are slightly apart though a little rounded (like a tube).
   b. The jaw (mandible) is lowered in the back (low mandible maneuver [LMM], second strategy).
   c. The tongue tip may be at the lower front teeth or a little raised. The blade and body of the tongue are depressed, creating a groove along the midline; the tongue edges make contact with the upper gum ridge.
   d. The velopharyngeal port is closed.

e. The vocal folds are together (adducted), hence creating sound.

f. The airstream is channeled through the groove in the tongue and breaks against the upper gum ridge (alveolar ridge) and front teeth, creating turbulence.

2. Step-by-step instructions

The /z/ consovowel (pitch + noise) may seem simple and may be the most frequent occurring fricative in the English language (Edwards, 2003). But it is also among the most difficult, and speech-language pathologists spend countless hours trying to correct this speech sound error. Non-native speakers of American English do not usually have a problem with it.

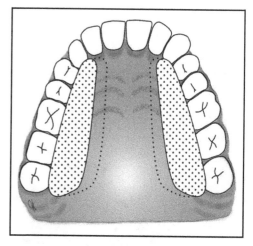

Figure 13–3. Contact of tongue edges with the upper gum ridge for /z/.

- Round your lips and place the tip of the tongue (apex) on the lower front teeth.
- Put your fingers on the joint that connects the jaw to your skull (temporomandibular joint [TMJ]). You can find that hinge in front of each ear (see Chapter 2, Figure 2–4).
- Drop the back of the jaw (posterior mandible) in a relaxed manner and feel in your fingers how the bone (condyle) moves forward and bulges. Your larynx will also relax downward (LMM, second strategy, Chapter 3), creating room in the pharynx.
- Depress the front blade of the tongue to a groove, imagining a depression of the genioglossus (see images in the preamble to Part II) as if you were holding a little bolus of water. With the groove, the tongue tip will retract, moving away and a little up from the lower teeth. For more help on the groove, have a look at Chapter 4.
- Once you create the groove, you will feel the edges on the upper gum ridge more prominently back to front (Figure 13–3). Should you not feel them

in the front or at all, you may have dropped the jaw too far.

- Take a breath and feel the cold air in that groove and around the edges of your teeth.
- With the /z/, sustain on a pitch while channeling the airstream along the center groove line of your tongue against the teeth. Notice the vibrations (which are the reflections of the sound within the oral cavity) behind the teeth, gum ridge (alveolar ridge) on the tongue surface, as well as the friction of the turbulence from the narrow constriction between teeth and tongue tip.
- Make sure the back of the tongue is relaxed and not trying to push toward the action in the front. And remember to let physics work for you (feel the pressure and airflow going backward, preventing the larynx and tongue from tensing up).

Common Challenges

Similar to the /ð/ fricative, sustaining on a "noisy" pitch can often be a challenge. The airstream is channeled centrally through the groove of the tongue, striking against the surface of the teeth, which can be quite loud at first. Subsequently, this may evoke a subconscious reaction to reduce the airflow and "fall back" into the larynx, pushing the laryngeal muscles to only "hold" the pitch so the noise does not "disturb" the sound. I often say, "don't make the /z/ too pretty by only phonating the pitch; the noise is part of the consovowel's identity."

Although the voiced nature of the /z/ phoneme does not require the same force as its voiceless cognate /s/, spreading of the lips as an instinctual counteraction to increase the airflow can always occur (Figure 13–4). The lip rounding in combination with the tongue guidance (groove) will help funnel the airstream with all its energy to the center of the teeth and not spread it to the side, losing power and lower frequencies. It helps to put your index fingers in the corner of the lips to help counteract the spreading.

The LMM can be another obstacle. Not lowering and relaxing the jaw (mandible)

and concomitantly the back of the tongue will reduce the space in the pharynx and push the tongue mass forward (making the space in the front even narrower and without a groove). As a result, the lower frequencies are being canceled out (pharyngeal constriction), and the higher frequencies are scattered and weak (a missing groove).

Last, but not least, we mention the tip of the tongue (apex): As mentioned in the general considerations, in fricatives we do not push the tongue tip (apex) against the upper gum ridge (alveolar) or teeth for that matter. We have to maintain a precise tongue shape, particularly the tip, in close proximity to the lower teeth. It is possible that efforts to either make the groove or maintain the position and shape may be initiated by the tongue tip, making it curl too much. This takes away the higher frequencies and, as you will see in our next consonant, modifies the phoneme from /z/ to a more /ʒ/-like phoneme, as in "pleasure."

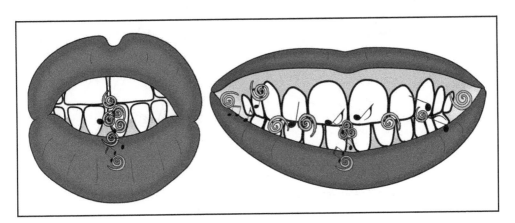

Figure 13–4. Relaxed, round lips (*left*) versus spread lips (*right*) for /z/.

/ʒ/ as in Plea<u>s</u>ure

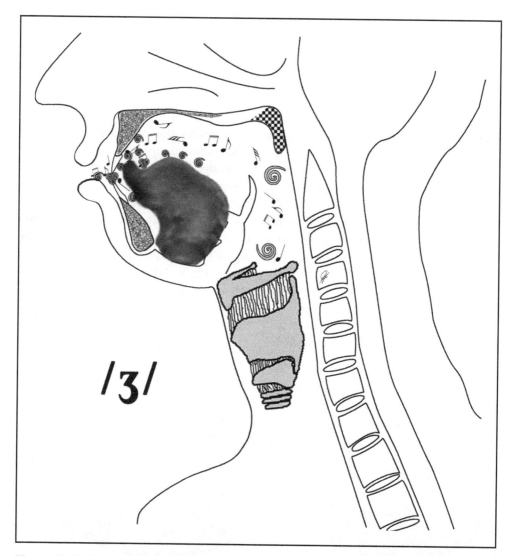

Figure 13–5. Ultrasound representation of /ʒ/.

Articulatory Considerations

1. Physiological description
   a. The lips are slightly apart, rounded, and protruded.
   b. The jaw (mandible) is lowered in the back (LMM, second strategy).
   c. The tongue tip (apex) is curled. The blade and body of the tongue are depressed, creating a groove along the midline; the tongue edges make contact with the upper gum ridge.
   d. The velopharyngeal port is closed.

e. The vocal folds are together (abducted), hence creating sound.

f. The airstream is channeled through the groove in the tongue, and turbulence results as it passes against the gum ridge, palate, and front teeth.

2. Step-by-step instructions

The /ʒ/ is one of the most acoustically powerful fricatives. It may have similarities with the /s/, although as the ultrasound clearly shows, it does have a distinct difference.

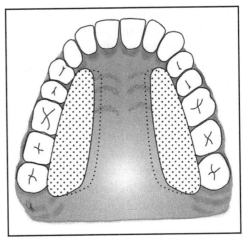

Figure 13–6. Contact of tongue edges with the upper gum ridge for /ʒ/.

- Round your lips and place the tip of your tongue (apex) against the lower front teeth.
- Put your fingers on the joint that connects the jaw to your skull (TMJ). You can find that hinge in front of each ear (see Chapter 2, Figure 2–4).
- Drop the back of the jaw (posterior mandible) in a relaxed manner and feel in your fingers how the bone (condyle) moves forward and bulges. Your larynx will also relax downward (LMM, second strategy, Chapter 3), creating room in the pharynx.
- Depress the front of the blade of the tongue to form a groove, imagining a depression of the genioglossus (see images in the preamble to Part II) as if you are holding a little bolus of water. With the groove, retract and curl the tongue tip upward, toward the gum ridge (alveolar). For more help on the groove, have a look at Chapter 4.
- Once you create the groove, you will feel the edges on the upper gum ridge more prominently back to front (Figure 13–6). Should you not feel them in the front or at all, you may have dropped the jaw too far.
- Take a breath and feel the cold air stroking the tip of the tongue and around the edges of your teeth.

- With the /ʒ/, sustain on a pitch, channeling the airstream along the centered groove of your tongue, against the upper palate and teeth. Notice the vibration (which is the reflection of the sound within the oral cavity) behind the teeth, gum ridge (alveolar ridge)/palate, and on the tongue surface, as well as the friction of the turbulence from the narrow constriction between teeth.
- And finally, make sure the back of the tongue is relaxed and does not push toward the action in the front. As always, let physics work for you (feel the pressure and airflow going backward, preventing the larynx and tongue from tensing up).

Common Challenges

Sometimes, the curling of the tongue tip itself, or keeping it in close proximity to the palate can be challenging. To make it easier, I suggest you first make contact with the palate (sealing it like a stop consonant), heightening the awareness of the position of the tip of your tongue. Next, build up the pressure behind it and feel the increase in the oral cavity through the expansion of the walls in the vocal tract, and particularly on the surface of the tongue (like expanding the groove). Also, make sure to keep everything centered and not pushed sideways. Next, release the tip from the palate, opening just a little bit, and notice the hizzing sound (higher fequencies) created by the air jet passing through the narrow constriction, breaking against the gum ridge and teeth. Basically, we just made a /dʒ/ (as in ju<u>dge</u>), which is phonating /d/ and /ʒ/ in close succession. Toggle back and forth between the two and notice the little movement necessary for the tip of the tongue to release and, importantly, how close in proximity it stays to the palate. Once you are comfortable with the movement, leave the /d/ out and only sustain on the /ʒ/. Of course, with all the attention focused on the front of the mouth, the jaw and back of the tongue may have become stiff and need to relax again (see earlier).

As with the cognate /ʃ/, spreading of the lips as an instinctual counteraction to increase the airflow can always occur (see Figure 13–4). The lip rounding in combination with the tongue guidance (groove) will help funnel the airstream with all its energy to the center of the teeth and not spread it to the side, losing power and lower frequencies. It helps to put your index fingers in the corner of the lips to help counteract the spreading.

The LMM can be another obstacle. Not lowering and relaxing the jaw (mandible) and concomitantly the back of the tongue will reduce the space in the pharynx and push the tongue mass forward (making the space in the front even narrower and without groove). As a result, the lower frequencies are being canceled out (pharyngeal constriction), and the higher frequencies are scattered and weak (missing groove).

Finally, concomitant with that, more often than not, tension emanates in the larynx in order to "create" the noise part of the consonant or reduce it because it is too loud (as with the /z/). Changing the airflow through various constrictions along our vocal tract will change the pressure within the mouth and vocal folds (glottis). For instance, a constriction in the front, as in the /ʒ/, will increase the pressure in the mouth (oral pressure) but decrease the pressure at the vocal folds (transglottal pressure), and vice versa. This is why we always want to be as efficient as possible and let physics work for us. The tongue tip between the teeth forms a constriction that in turn creates friction, which is the noise part associated with the consonant. Hence, there is no need to separately add any musculature action by pushing harder, particularly not from the throat. This would not only make it harder for the vocal folds to maintain vibration (oscillation) but also reduce the necessary pressure for the constriction in the front. Envisioning the airflow going backward into the mouth will help prevent the upward push in the larynx and keep the balance of the vocal folds' vibration and the constriction between tongue front and teeth.

/v/ as in <u>V</u>ine

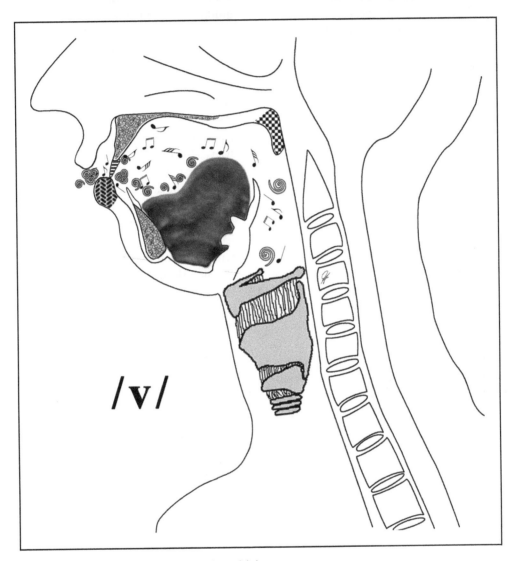

Figure 13–7. Ultrasound representation of /v/.

Articulatory Considerations

1. Physiological description
   a. The jaw (mandible) is lowered in the back (LMM, second strategy).
   b. The inner border of the lower lip is slightly rounded and raised to contact the upper teeth.
   c. The tongue tip (apex) may touch the lower jaw ridge on the bottom of the mouth behind the lower

teeth. The blade and body of the tongue are depressed, creating a groove along the midline.

d. The velopharyngeal port is closed.
e. The vocal folds are together (abducted), hence creating sound.
f. The airstream is channeled along the groove through the light closure of the lower lip and upper teeth, thus creating friction.

2. Step-by-step instructions

The outgoing airflow creates a friction noise because of the constriction lip-teeth (labio-dental) obstruction. But, as always, we have to start with building the resonance around it.

- Put your fingers on the joint that connects the jaw to your skull (TMJ). You can find that hinge in front of each ear (see Chapter 2, Figure 2–4).
- Drop the back of the jaw (posterior mandible) in a relaxed manner and feel in your fingers how the bone (condyle) moves forward and bulges. Your larynx will also relax downward (LMM, second strategy, Chapter 3), creating room in the pharynx.
- Set the vowel /ɑ/, depress the front blade of the tongue to a groove; imagine a depression of the genioglossus (see images in the preamble to Part II) as if you were holding a little scoop of ice cream that you do not want to touch your teeth. For more help on the groove, have a look at Chapter 4. The tongue tip may touch the lower jaw ridge on the bottom of the mouth behind the lower teeth. The back of the tongue elongates with the second strategy of the LMM.
- Take a breath and slightly protrude both upper and lower lips. Raise the slightly more rounded and protruded

lower lip to make contact with its inner border and upper teeth.
- With the /v/, sustain on a pitch while guiding the airstream along the centered groove of your tongue to the middle of the place of articulation. Notice the vibrations (which are the reflections of the sound within the oral cavity) behind the teeth (or even within them), the gum ridge (alveolar ridge)/palate, and on the tongue surface, as well as the friction of the turbulence from the narrow constriction between the lower lip and incisors.
- Feel the backpressure from the small and constricted outlet in the front and let physics work for you. To prevent tension in your tongue and larynx, envision the airflow going backward into the mouth, and make sure the back of the tongue is relaxed and does not push toward the action in the front.

Common Challenges

We have already seen that noise generated by friction alone would make a very weak acoustic signal. Ensuring maximum consonant resonance with the tongue shaping the vowel /ɑ/, applying the LMM (Chapter 3), and adding a pitch (vocal fold vibration) has been shown to provide good acoustic power to this consovowel (noise + pitch, Chapter 7).

As in our previous consonant, it is not uncommon that simultaneously with the lip spreading, tension emanates in the larynx in order to "create" the noise part of the consonant or reduce it because it may be too loud. Spreading the lips as an instinctive counteraction to increase the airflow will weaken the acoustic power (Figure 13–8). To bal-

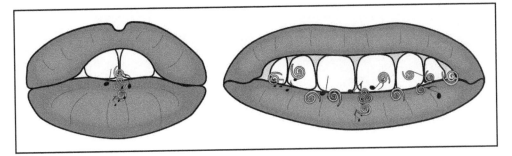

Figure 13–8. Relaxed, round lips (*left*) versus spread lips (*right*) for /v/.

ance the increased pressure in the front (due to the constriction) with the decreased pressure in between the vocal folds (transglottal pressure), we let physics work for us. The incisors with the inner border of the lower lip form a constriction that in turn creates friction, which is the noise part associated with the consonant. Hence, there is no need to separately add any muscular action by pushing harder, particularly not from the throat. This would not only make it harder for the vocal folds to maintain vibration (oscillation) but also reduce the necessary pressure for the constriction in the front. Envisioning the airflow going backward into the mouth will help prevent the upward push in the larynx and keep the balance of the vocal folds' vibration and the constric-

tion between tongue front and teeth. The lip rounding in combination with the tongue guidance (groove) will help funnel the airstream with all its energy to the center of the teeth and not spread it to the side. It helps to put your index fingers in the corner of the lips to help counteract the spreading. It will also help prevent the cheeks from puffing up, which would also be an indicator of losing the energy to the side.

Reference

Edwards, H. T. (2003). *Applied phonetics: The sounds of American English* (3rd ed.). Clifton Park, NY: Thomson.

14 Rhotic, Non-English R-Sounds—/ř/ /ɾ/ /ʁ/

General Considerations

Recall that the schwa forms /ɚ/ (as in mother) and /ɝ/ (as in earth) are covered in Chapter 6, considering them as vowels. Among phoneticians, the classification and description of the English /r/ are quite ambiguous. As a tenet of maximum consonant resonance (CR) on stage, singers and actors may prefer to think of this phoneme as a full vowel.

Before we continue, a note regarding the use of the International Phonetic Alphabet (IPA) symbols is in order. The IPA provides a variety of "r" symbols, starting from plain, rotated to otherwise modified versions of the letter "r." The symbol of /r/ is usually assigned to the rolled "r," though phoneticians have also adapted it for the generic vowel-like English "r." In this book, we join the latter, using /r/ for the English "r" and adapting the use of the wedge /ˇ/ above the /r/—so it appears as /ř/—for the rolled "r" to indicate the physical activity of the tongue tip (G. Nair, 1999).

There are two kinds of /r/ in English usage:

- ▪ "r" that functions almost like a glide, and
- ▪ "r" that is actually a rhotic vowel.

The technical dividing line between the two usages is tongue movement or stability: R as an on- or off-glide in combination with a vowel (the discrete /r/). Say the words listed in Table 14–1 (Edwards, 2003).

Each of these usages either initiates or releases a vowel and involves a shift of the tongue between the two phonemes. Examples of rhotic vowel forms are listed in Table 14–2 (Edwards, 2003).

In each of these examples, there is no discrete tongue shift between the vowel

Table 14–1. Example of Discrete /r/

rabbit	ræbɪt
carrot	kæɾət
car	kɑr
wrench	rɛntʃ
peril	peɾəl
star	stɑr

Table 14–2. Examples of Rhotic Vowel Forms

earth	ɝθ
bird	bɝd
herb	ɝb
curtain	kɝtən
spur	spɝr

and the /r/. In effect, the vowel combines with the /r/ as a rhotic and is executed with a stable tongue. During the syllable in which the /r/ occurs in those words, the tongue does not move. Tongue *motion* or *stability* is the differentiating condition between the two.

There are not many languages of this world that possess the American English vowel-like /r/ sound (Edwards, 2003). Although a quite frequent sound in English, it is rather a difficult one to master not only for children or non-native speakers but, ironically enough, also for English native actors and singers. Most word-interior rhotic vowels must be written as stressed schwar (e.g., mother /mʌðɚ/). In Chapter 6, we saw how minimal the movements for the "r" in the schwa forms are, and similar to the fricatives, we do not have an articulator holding against another. In other words, we only have a precise tongue shape held for a noticeable period of time (stability).

Additionally, contextualization (sociolinguistics) not only shows itself in the use of language and discourse to signal relevant aspects of an interactional or communicative situation (e.g., informal style "kinda" versus formal style "kind of"), but it also changes the pitch, resonance, and, particularly, articulation. In a setting like the stage, TV, or presentation, it is not uncommon to find people rightfully concerned about their enunciation. However, in doing so, they find themselves lost in the phonetics of their own language because they may never have looked at it through that perspective.

Remember the building blocks of language in Chapter 5? Sometimes we are unaware of the sounds of our own language and, as in English, confuse the letters of the alphabet with the sound of the language. Let us assume that an actor wants to sustain on the first two letters of "great" to convey his enthusiasm. However, because the /g/ is a prevoiced stop, the /r/ is the only phoneme of the two that he can elongate. Without wanting it to sound like a /ɻ/ (retroflex) or "hard r," he would need to maintain (stability) just a little curl of the tip of the tongue near the lower teeth instead of the full back curl of the /ɻ/ (Figure 14–1). This is similar to that we have seen with the /z/ and /ʒ/ (Chapter 13). Remember, changing the filter (tongue, jaw, etc.) will change the source (sound), as discussed in Chapter 5. As mentioned earlier, the tongue motion and/or stability is the differentiating condition between the two.

Actors and singers must avoid the use of the retroflex-r, unless the *characterization* of a role demands its dialectal use. One more note regarding the "r" pronunciation in the context of music: There is always the debate over whether its traditional sung pronunciation, such as in Handel's *Messiah*, has been a rolled /ř/, flipped /ɾ/, or discrete English /r/. Thanks to research by musicologists and musicians, we know a lot about historical performance practice, and there is a lot of literature on how to pronounce Latin in classical singing (German style, Italian style, etc.), yet the literature on how to pronounce the English texts seems to be insufficient.

It seems to me that over the past decades, recordings of well-known professional singers, choirs and conductors worldwide have established an unquestioned tradition with no linguistic basis—the use of /ř/ (rolled "r") for anything English. Of course, one could argue that Handel was a German, and that prestige British English of the 18th century was more rhotic, or at least flipped (/ɾ/), although even linguists are still not certain about that. *Note:* for the reader who is interested in digging deeper into the history of English pronunciation, I recommend starting with Dobson's, *English Pronunciation* (1985), Strang's, *A History of English* (2015), and Beal's *English in Modern Times* (2014).

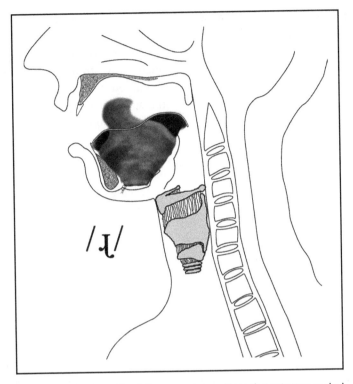

Figure 14–1. Retroflex /ɻ/ tongue shape. Note the extreme curled tongue tip (apex) creating a highly concave tongue shape. For comparison, the vocalic /r/ (/ɐ/) indicated by the tongue shape (*black/yellow*) and surface (*white/red*).

However, as in our earlier example, as singers we want to have good resonance, diction, and expression of the text. So, to accomplish all of it, singers tend to exaggerate the English /r/ by unwittingly using the /ɻ/ (retroflex). Unfortunately, the extreme tongue position translates into stiffness of the tongue and larynx, compromising CR, overall sound, and authentic pronunciation. The popular solution to this problem seems to be the complete opposite: the /r̆/ (rolled "r"). However, this would be creating a problem in order to solve a problem. Having the patience to teach how to actually sustain on the vowel-like English /r/—that is, maintaining the tongue stability—may help with the excessive trills, though it would also require the knowledge to do so.

Of course, in an aria such as "The trumpet shall sound" (from Handel's *Messiah*), the singer may want to impart some excitement by lightly trilling on the "r," though not anywhere near an Italian /r̆/.

The same excessive use of the /r̆/ can be found in German. Here too, some of it is partially driven by incredible singers such as the great Dietrich Fischer-Dieskau. He may have overused the /r̆/ (rolled) at the beginning of his career, up until around the 1950s, but he started increasing the vocalic /ɐ/ after that. Unfortunately, others did not, and it seems that in the classical singing world, change does not happen at the same pace as it does in speech. We already talked about the history of the rules for "standard/ high German" (sometimes also referred to as *Bühnenaussprache* [stage language], Chapter 11). According to the Duden *Das Aussprachewörterbuch,* we find the following rules:

/ř/ (rolled)

→ *before syllabic[1] and nonsyllabic vowels:* (Rat /řaːt/ = advise; zerren /tsɛřən/ = to drag; Zahnrad / tsaːnřaːt/ = gear).

→ *After short vowels (/ɪ ɛ ʏ œ a ʊ ɔ/) at the end of a word or before a consonant:* (gern /gɛřn/ = gladly; Irrtum /ɪřtuːm/ = mistake).

/ɐ/ (vocalic)

→ *After the long vowel /aː/ (similar to "up") or before a consonant:* (Haar / haːɐ/ = hair; Harz /haːɐts/ = resin).

→ *After the long vowels /i: e: ɛ: y: ø: u: o:/:* (hört /høɐt/ = sb. Hears; fährst / fɛɐst/ = drive).

However, these rules come with two big caveats: (a) certain regional influences may change the pronunciation of the /ř/ to /ɐ/, and vice versa; and (b) the transformation of the spoken /r/ in German has also influenced the artistic use of the /r/ in classical singing. As with the German *ich*-laut /ç/ (discussed in Chapter 11), an IPA's transliteration of a local dialect might be accurate yet may violate the rules presented earlier. Furthermore, we are trying to envision a purer and more standardized language where we want to incorporate more "modernized" pronunciation patterns. The latter is of particular interest, because as artists we tend to unquestioningly adapt and follow our idols and mentors with big names. While there is nothing wrong with that, we ought to be careful what we implement and as with our ich-Laut /ç/, ask ourselves about the authenticity and correctness of today's pronunciation. Over the past two decades, numerous authors of singing books have started to follow this evolution of the international consensus. An article in *Journal of Singing* by Wencke Ophaug skillfully summarizes the development of the use of different /r/-variants in the German lied, and presents a set of rules of today's usage of /r/-allophones in the German classical (Ophaug, 2010).

One of the main tenets of this book involves the use of CR to invoke proper vocal performance. Being able to discern and execute between the subtle differences of tongue motion and stability is the foundation for continuous vocal resonance, intelligibility, and artistic freedom. The French socialist Jean Jaurès once responded to conservative congressmen, "*Tradition ist die Weitergabe des Feuers und nicht die Anbetung der Asche*" (Tradition is the handing down of the flame and not the worshipping of ashes) (Krieghofer, 2017). Continuing a certain form of pronunciation because it is a tradition certainly is an artistic right. However, doing so because of lack of technique, knowledge, or as Jaurès continued to say, "because of coziness and laziness" would be a betrayal of artistic integrity. All performing arts recognize techniques and standards that also evolve over time, just like the changes in pronunciation of the German /r/ (and also in several other languages) seen over several decades.

---

[1]The vowel or vowel-like consonant that forms a syllable on its own.

/ř/ as in *Rapporto* (Italian for "Report")

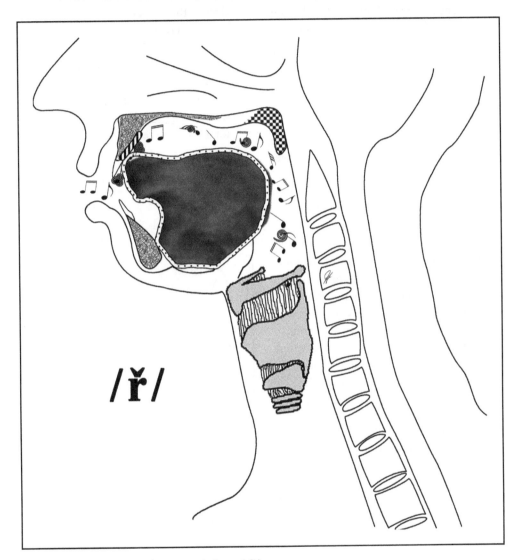

/ř/

Figure 14–2. Ultrasound representation of /ř/.

Articulatory Considerations

1. Physiological description
   a. The lips are apart though a little rounded (like a tube).
   b. The jaw (mandible) is lowered in the back (low mandible maneuver [LMM], second strategy).
   c. The tip of the tongue vibrates (indicated by white dotted/red outline) against the upper teeth or gum ridge (alveolar). The blade and body of the tongue are depressed, creating a groove along the midline; the tongue edges contact the upper gum ridge.

d. The velopharyngeal port is closed.
e. The vocal folds are together (adducted), hence creating sound.
f. The airstream is channeled through the groove in the tongue, evoking the Bernoulli effect between the tip of the tongue and the gum ridge (alveolar).

2. Step-by-step instructions

The rolled /ř/ consovowel (pitch + noise, Chapter 7) is quite difficult and may need a lot of practice to master.

▨ With the mouth comfortably open, find contact with the tip of the tongue behind the upper teeth. The tongue sides are sealing off the oral cavity along the upper gum ridge (Figure 14–3). Breathing should only be possible through the mouth (oral cavity).

▨ Along with the previous instructions, the front blade of the tongue depresses to a groove. Imagine a depression of the genioglossus (see images in the preamble to Part II) as if you would hold a little bolus of water. With the groove, the sealing along the upper gum ridge may move a little inward.

▨ Once you sealed off the entire oral cavity, release the tip of the tongue while maintaining contact with the edges of the tongue.

▨ The lips may be a little protruded, like a tube, which will prevent them from spreading and help balance out the turbulences (Figure 14–4).

▨ With the /ř/ sustained on a pitch and sufficient airflow, channel the air jet along the centered groove line of the

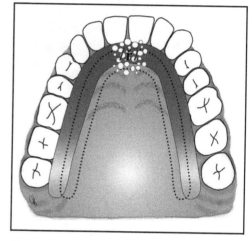

Figure 14–3. Range of place of articulation (PoA) for /ř/. Turbulence and flapping at the tip of the tongue (*white/blue circles*).

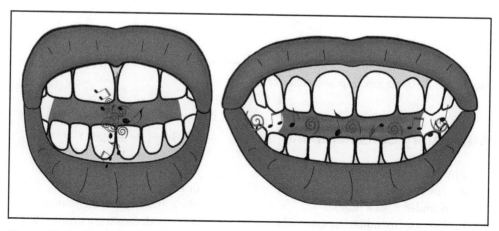

Figure 14–4. Consovowel /ř/: relaxed, puckered lips (*left*) versus spread lips (*right*).

tongue to start the rapid flutter of the tip of the tongue. Notice the vibration and noise created by the repeating patterns of the closing and opening of the flow channel.

▪ Remember to let physics work for you. Imagine the airflow going backward, preventing the larynx and tongue from tensing up and pushing the tip of the tongue against the teeth.

Common Challenges

This consovowel (pitch + noise, Chapter 7) poses a big challenge for a lot of people, and not only those with ankyloglossia (tongue-tie). If the rolled-r /ř/ does not come naturally, it will require careful practice and a lot of patience. As always, at the beginning it is about creating awareness. Starting with a /d/ (as in d̲og) has proven to be a good way to begin that process because the tongue sealing off the front of the oral cavity in the /d/ is virtually the same configuration as that for the /ř/.

Begin by setting the tongue for the /d/ (see Chapter 10), build up the pressure but hold off with the release. Instead, slowly start to move the tip of the tongue down and up, releasing air in increments, like a valve turning water on and off. If the tongue starts to flutter, increase the pressure, particularly in the mouth, to maintain it for as long as possible. The goal is to gradually increase the time to sustain the flutter with every attempt.

Here is where our "let physics work for you" comes into play. The strike of the tip of the tongue against the gum ridge (alveola) creates the characteristic noise associated with this consonant. Hence, there is no need to separately add to that by pushing harder, particularly not from the throat. The image of picturing the force of the airflow going backward into the mouth is preventing the tension in the larynx and helps to balance sufficient air pressure as well as the tensegrity (tension and integrity, discussed in Chapter 2) of the tongue.

Similar to the /ð/ fricative, sustaining on a "noisy" pitch can often be a challenge. The airstream is channeled centrally through the groove of the tongue, striking against the surface of the teeth, which can be quite loud at first. Subsequently, this may evoke a subconscious reaction to reduce the airflow and "fall back" into the larynx, pushing the laryngeal muscles to only "hold" the pitch so the noise does not "disturb" the sound. I often say, "don't make the /z/ too pretty by only phonating the pitch; the noise is part of the consovowel's identity."

Although the voiced nature of the /ř/ phoneme does not require the same force as voiceless /s/, for instance, spreading of the lips as an instinctual counteraction to increase the airflow can always occur (see Figure 14–3). The lip rounding in combination with the tongue guidance (groove) will help funnel the airstream with all its energy to the center of the teeth and not spread it to the side, losing power and lower frequencies. It helps to put your index fingers in the corners of your lips to help counteract the spreading.

/r/ as in *Ador̲o* (Italian for "I Love")

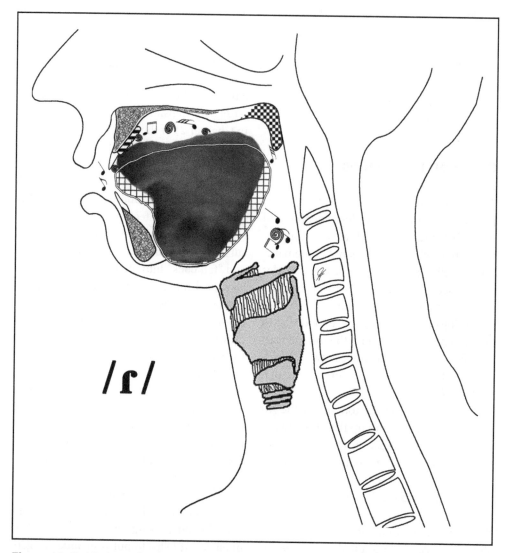

Figure 14–5. Ultrasound representation of /r/.

Articulatory Considerations

1. Physiological description
   a. The lips are apart though a little rounded (like a tube).
   b. The jaw (mandible) is lowered in the back (LMM, second strategy).
   c. The tip of the tongue vibrates against the upper teeth or gum ridge (alveolar) once or twice (the white squared/green outline indicates the position following release after contact). The blade and body of the tongue are depressed, creat-

ing a groove along the midline; the tongue edges contact the upper gum ridge.

d. The velopharyngeal port is closed.

e. The vocal folds are together (adducted), hence creating sound.

f. The airstream is channeled through the groove in the tongue, evoking the Bernoulli effect between the tip of the tongue and the gum ridge (alveolar).

2. Step-by-step instructions

The flipped-r (/ɾ/) is executed like the rolled-r (/r̆/), except for the number of contacts. Instead of a continuous flutter, the tip of the tongue contacts the gum ridge (alveolar) only once or twice.

▢ With the mouth comfortably open, find contact with the tip of the tongue behind the upper teeth. The sides of the tongue are sealing off the oral cavity along the upper gum ridge (Figure 14–6). Breathing should only be possible through the mouth (oral cavity).

▢ Along with the previous instructions, the front blade of the tongue depresses to a groove. Imagine a depression of the genioglossus (see images in the preamble to Part II) as if holding a little bolus of water. With the groove, the sealing along the upper gum ridge may move a little inward.

▢ Once you have sealed off the entire oral cavity, release the tip of the tongue while maintaining contact with the edges of the tongue.

▢ The lips may be a little protruded, like a tube, which will prevent them from spreading and help balance out the turbulence (see Figure 14–4).

▢ With the /ɾ/ and on a pitch, channel the air jet along the centered groove line of the tongue to single or double strike the tip of the tongue against the gum ridge (alveolar). Notice how the one-two strikes of the tip of the tongue against the gum ridge create the noise part of the consovowel.

▢ Remember to let physics work for you. Imagine the airflow going backward, preventing the larynx and tongue from tensing up and pushing the tip of the tongue against the teeth.

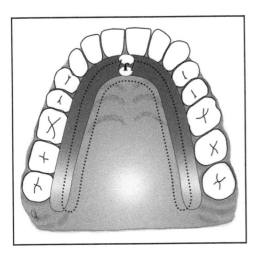

Figure 14–6. Range of place of articulation (PoA) for /ɾ/. Turbulence and short flap (one-two) at the tip of the tongue (*white/blue circles*).

Common Challenges

As mentioned earlier, the flipped-r /ɾ/ is similar to the rolled /r̆/, only now we have a single short closure. Using the /d/ (as in <u>d</u>og), which has virtually the same configuration as that for the /ɾ/, will also help to begin that process of creating awareness in the tip of the tongue. So, set the tongue for the /d/ (described in Chapter 10) and build up the pressure, but hold off with the release. Instead, slowly start to move the tip of the tongue down and up, releasing air in increments, like a valve turning water on and off. Now, if the pressure in the mouth (interoral pressure) is too low, it may sound more like a /d/. If the tongue starts to flutter more than twice, try to cut off the airflow earlier rather than decreasing the pressure.

Here is where our "let physics work for you" comes into play. The strike of the tip of the tongue against the gum ridge (alveola) creates the characteristic noise associated with this consonant. Hence, there is no need to add to any of that by pushing harder, particularly not from the throat. Also, it is a fine line between too much and too little air pressure, particularly in the mouth (interoral). Picture the force of the airflow going backward into the mouth, preventing the tension in the larynx and helping to balance sufficient air pressure as well as the tenseg-

rity (tension and integrity; see Chapter 2) of the tongue.

Last, but not least, do not forget the LMM. Put your fingers on the joint that connects the jaw to your skull (temporo-mandibular joint [TMJ]). You can find that hinge in front of each ear. Drop the back of the jaw (posterior mandible) in a relaxed manner and feel in your fingers how the bone (condyle) moves forward and bulges. Your larynx will also relax downward (LMM, second strategy, Chapter 3), creating room in the pharynx. This will help to relax the back of the tongue and increase the space in the pharynx as well as in the front, allowing enough space and proper angle for the tip of the tongue to move freely and not push the entire mass of the tongue forward.

/ʁ/ as in *Rouge* (French for "Red")

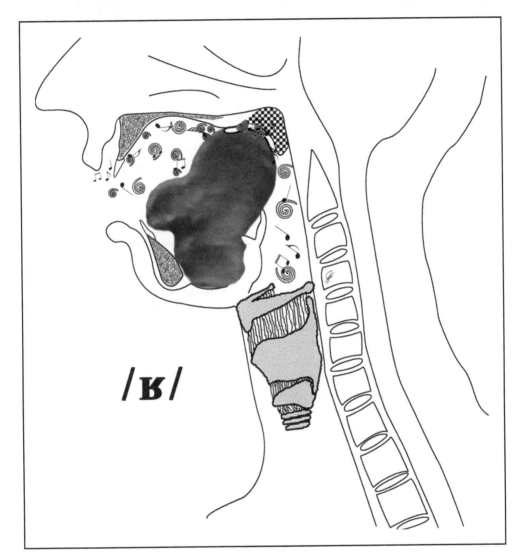

Figure 14–7. Ultrasound representation of /ʁ/.

Articulatory Considerations

1. Physiological description
   a. The lips are apart and neutral.
   b. The tongue body is raised to create a contact with the uvula.
   c. The velopharyngeal port is closed.
   d. The vocal folds are together (adducted), hence creating sound.
   e. Air goes through the constricting narrow channel of the tongue and uvula (PoA), causing turbulence that creates the noise associated with the phoneme.

2. Step-by-step instructions

Although this consovowel (pitch + noise, see Chapter 7) cannot be found in American English, as singers, one has to sing in many other languages. And as actors/actresses, one may have to mimic the sound for various reasons (e.g., dialect, scream, etc.).

- With the mouth still closed, put your fingers on the joint that connects the jaw to your skull (TMJ). You can find that hinge in front of each ear (pictured in Chapter 2, Figure 2–5).
- Without pushing it, drop the jaw as far as you can in a relaxed manner and feel in your fingers how the bone (condyle) moves forward and bulges. Your larynx will also relax downward.

Now focus your attention on your tongue.

- Allow the root of the tongue to relax (downward) as well, so it can elongate its trunk (see ultrasound image).
- Move the body along the hard palate back to the soft palate/velum and find the spot (PoA) that makes the relaxation/drop of the trunk/back of the tongue and jaw easier (Figure 14–8).
- Feel the contact of the tongue surface with the velum and imagine letting go of any tension in the trunk of the tongue to allow it to elongate (see ultrasound image). Also, keep the tip of the tongue low and prevent it from curling up, which would prevent the rest of the tongue body from forming.
- If you are still feeling a lot of tension, reset. But before you start again, bite on the edges of your tongue, and once you set the PoA again, imagine releasing those edges.
- Once you are set again, prepare for a sufficient airflow, and on a pitch,

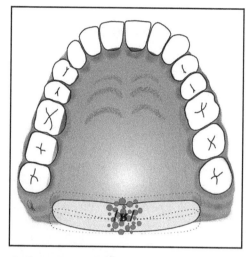

Figure 14–8. Possible places of articulation (PoA) for /ʁ/. Turbulence and flapping in the center of the tongue (*gray/blue circles*).

sustain the /ʁ/. Ideally, besides the pitch, you should hear a lot of white noise mixed with some low pulsating noise, almost like a trill. The latter is the uvula flapping against the tongue surface, which may need some time to actually start. It is somewhat like a reversed snore, only now the airstream is passing between only the uvula and tongue, rather than the uvula, tongue, and sinuses. In order to get a feel for it, you may want to experiment with this rather noisy exercise a little bit: Try to sniff back as if you want to clear your nose from congested mucus or simulate a snore and feel the flapping uvula. This will give you a sense of where the uvula is and what the turbulence between the constriction of the contact area feels like. Once you have established the sensation, try to replicate the same flapping for the consonant /χ/. As always, do not push it too hard, and imagine the direction going backward rather than outward.

Common Challenges

Ensuring maximum CR with the tongue shaping the vowel /ɑ/, applying the LMM (see Chapter 3), and adding a pitch (vocal fold vibration) has shown to provide good acoustic power to this consovowel (pitch + noise, see Chapter 7).

Spreading the lips as an instinctual counteraction to increase the airflow will also weaken the acoustic power (Figure 14–9). The lip rounding in combination with the tongue guidance (groove) will help funnel the airstream with all its energy to the center of the teeth and not spread it to the side, losing power and lower frequencies. It helps to put your index fingers in the corner of the lips to help counteract the spreading. It will also help prevent the cheeks from puffing up, which would also be an indicator of losing the energy to the side.

Concomitant with that, more often than not, tension emanates in the larynx in order to "create" the noise part of the consonant as well as the pitch. The flapping occurs because of the aerodynamic conditions: The back of the tongue is placed close enough to the uvula (a soft part), and an air jet of sufficient strength starts a repeating pattern of closing and opening. This is again a case where physics works for you. There is no need to add any musculature action such as pushing, particularly not from the throat. Imagining the airflow going backward into the mouth will help prevent the upward push in the larynx and keep the balance of the constriction between tongue and uvula. The same is true for the vocal folds. Adding the pitch to the noise does not need any actions from the muscles because a current of air of the right strength passing through them will initiate the phonation (opening and closing = oscillation).

Finally, do not forget the LMM. Put your fingers on the joint that connects the jaw to your skull (TMJ). You can find that hinge in front of each ear. Drop the back of the jaw (posterior mandible) in a relaxed manner and feel with your fingers how the bone (condyle) moves forward and bulges. Your larynx will also relax downward (LMM, second strategy, Chapter 3), creating room in the pharynx. This will help to relax the back of the tongue and increase the space

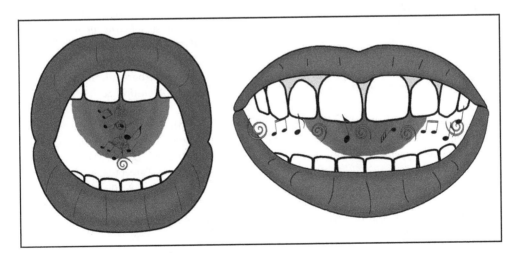

Figure 14–9. Consovowel /ʁ/: relaxed, little puckered lips (*left*) versus spread lips (*right*).

in the pharynx as well as in the front, allowing enough space and the proper angle for the tip of the tongue to move freely and not push the entire mass of the tongue forward. You may want to use a tongue depressor to help prevent the tip of tongue from curling upward (as described in Chapter 4), thus freeing the root of the tongue.

References

Beal, J. C. (2014). *English in modern times.* New York, NY: Routledge.

Dobson, E. J. (1985). *English pronunciation 1500–1700* (Vol. II). Oxford, UK: Clarendon Press.

Edwards, H. T. (2003). *Applied phonetics: The sounds of American English* (3rd ed.). Clifton Park, NY: Thomson.

Krieghofer, G. (2017) *Irrwege einer Metapher.* Wiener Zeitung.at http://www.wienerzeitung.at/themen_channel/wz_reflexionen/geschichten/897102_Irrwege-einer-Metapher.html

Nair, G. (1999). *Voice, tradition and technology.* San Diego, CA: Singular Publishing.

Ophoug, W. (2010). The pronunciation of /r/ in German classical singing. *Journal of Singing, 66*(5), 561–574.

Strang, B. M. H. (2015). *A history of English* (Vol. 26). New York, NY: Routledge.

Further Reading

Deme, A. (2014). Intelligibility of sung vowels: The effect of consonantal context and the onset of voicing. *Journal of Voice, 28*(4), 523. e19–523.e25

Fogerty, D., & Humes, L. E. (2012). The role of vowel and consonant fundamental frequency, envelope, and temporal fine structure cues to the intelligibility of words and sentences.
Journal of the Acoustical Society of America, 131(2), 1490–1501.

Gottfried, T. L., & Chew, S. L. (1986). Intelligibility of vowels sung by a countertenor. *Journal of the Acoustical Society of America, 79,* 124–130.

Gramming, P., Sundberg, J., Ternström, S., Leanderson, R., & Perkins, W. H. (1987). Relationship between changes in voice pitch and loudness. *STL-Quarterly Progress and Status Report, 28*(1), 39–55.

Gregg, J. W., & Scherer, R. C. (2005). Vowel intelligibility in classical singing. *Journal of Voice, 20*(2), 198–210.

Hollien, H., Mendes-Schwartz, A. P., & Nielsen, K. (2000). Perceptual confusions of high-pitched sung vowels. *Journal of Voice, 14,* 188–197.

Hunter, E. J., & Titze, I. (2010). Variations in intensity, fundamental frequency, and voicing for teachers in occupational versus non-occupational settings. *Journal of Speech, Language, and Hearing Research, 53*(4), 862–875.

Lee, S-H., Kwon, H-J., Choi, H-J., Lee, N-H., Lee, S-J., & Jin, S-M. (2008). The singer's formant and speaker's ring resonance: A long-term average spectrum analysis. *Clinical and Experimental Otorhinolaryngology, 1*(2), 92–96.

Miller, G. A., & Nicely, P. E. (1955). An analysis of perceptual confusions among some English consonants. *Journal of the Acoustical Society of America, 27,* 338–353.

Öhman, S. E. G. (1966). Coarticulation in VCV utterances: Spectrographic measurements. *Journal of the Acoustical Society of America, 39,* 151–168.

Rodet, X. (2008). Methods for singing voice control and synthesis. *Journal of the Acoustical Society of America, 123*(5), 3378.

Sundberg, J. (1994). Perceptual aspects of singing. *Journal of Voice, 8,* 106–122.

Sundberg, J., & Romedahl, C. (2009). Text intelligibility and the singer's formant—A relationship? *Journal of Voice, 23*(5), 539–545.

Titze, I. R. (1982). Why is the verbal message less intelligible in singing than in speech? *Journal of Singing, 38*(3), 37.

Welch, G. F., & Sundberg, J. (2002). Solo voice. In R. Parncutt & G. E. McPherson (Eds.), *The science and psychology of music performance: Creative strategies for teaching and learning* (pp. 253–268). New York, NY: Oxford University Press.

15 Affricates and Para-Affricates— /dz/ /dʒ/ /ts/ /tʃ/ /ks/

General Considerations

With this chapter, we are about to close the circle of the most frequent consonants one will encounter as an actor/singer. Only now, we are not looking at new consonants but rather combinations of consonants we already worked on. Thus, we only point out some general considerations and show the ultrasound sequence of each pair.

In general, an affricate is a compound consonant that begins as a stop and is released as a fricative. Have a look at the International Phonetic Alphabet (IPA). Until now, we covered a single symbol representing the sound of a given consonant. Now we look at two symbols. In English, only /dʒ/ (as in ju_dge_) and /tʃ/ (as in chur_ch_) are considered affricates among phoneticians. Yet, other combinations, such as /dz/ (as in o_dds_), /ts/ (as in ca_ts_), and /ks/ (as in xero_x_), can also be found. Even though they may not function as pure affricates, as singers and actors we want to look at them phonetically, and in that way, they do. For this reason, for the other combination phonemes we are going to adapt the term *para-affricates* from Garyth Nair (2007), where *para* means "to stand beside."

The challenges in the execution of affricates and para-affricates are the speed, length, and continuum of each of them. Most often, the fricative (consonant produced by constricting the vocal tract to produce turbulence) following the occlusion is extended as well as being voiced or voiceless. So, for instance, the fluctuation of pressure in the stop consonant has to be immediately managed by the following fricative. This time, we cannot keep a gap after the stop consonant (described in Chapter 9) to balance out the increased pressure. However, with both stop and aspiration or fricative phase being homorganic (same place of articulation [PoA]), maintaining a continuum should be easier. An exception is /ks/, where the PoAs are almost on opposite sides. If the location (PoA) and setup of point A (/k/) and point B (/s/) are not clear before their execution, the end result is most likely going to be a comic sound effect.

Reference

Nair, G. (2007). *The craft of singing*. San Diego, CA: Plural Publishing.

/dz/ as in O**dds**

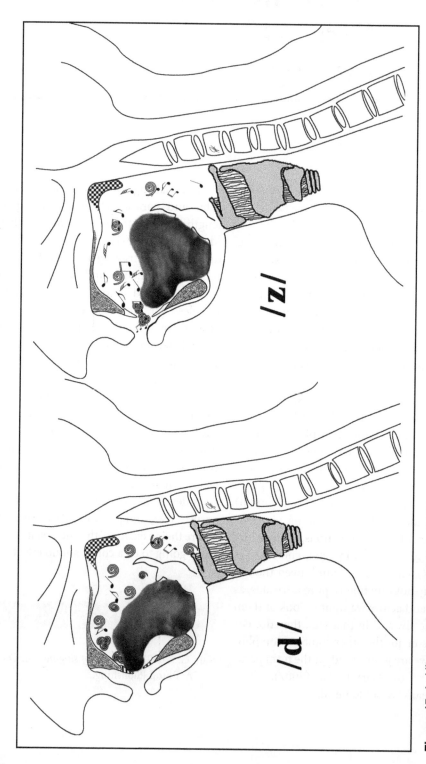

Figure 15–1. Ultrasound representation of /dz/.

/dʒ/ as in <u>J</u>u<u>dg</u>e

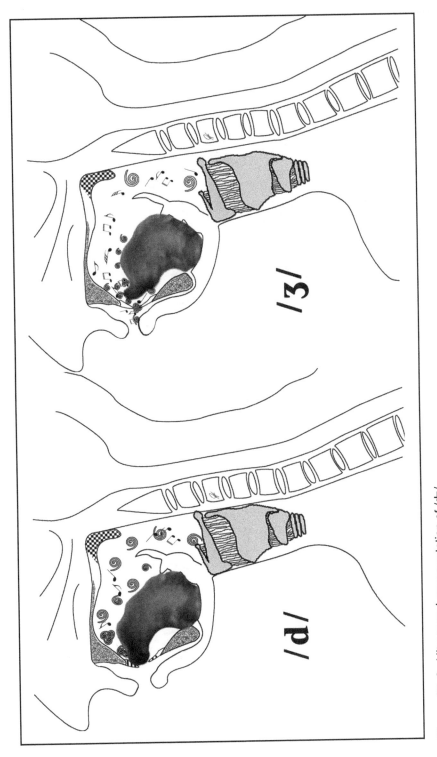

Figure 15–2. Ultrasound representation of /dʒ/.

/ts/ as in Cats

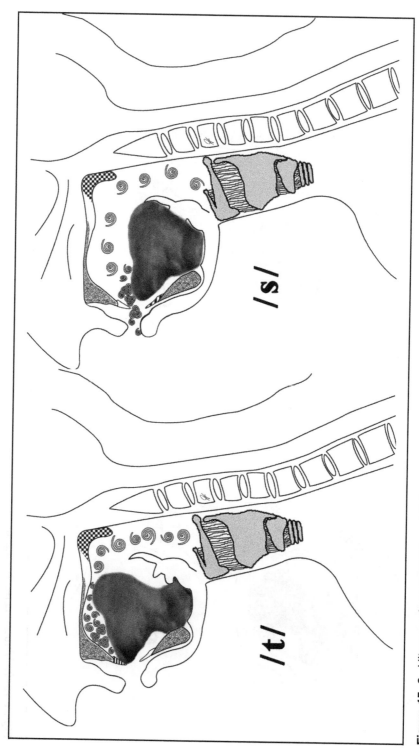

Figure 15–3. Ultrasound representation of /ts/.

/tʃ/ as in Catch

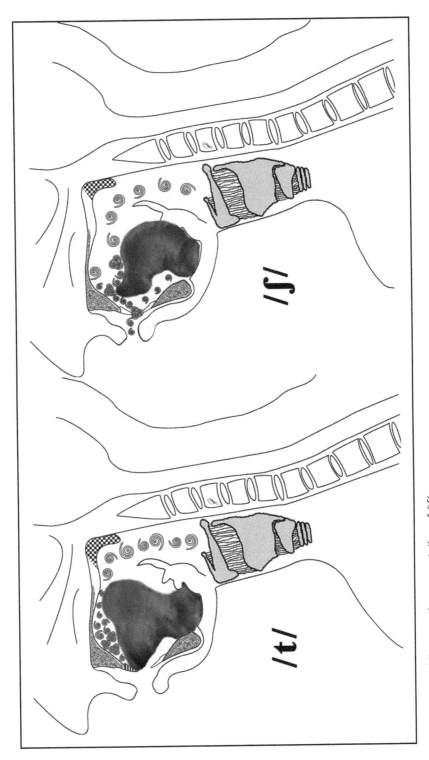

Figure 15–4. Ultrasound representation of /tʃ/.

/ks/ as in Xero<u>x</u>

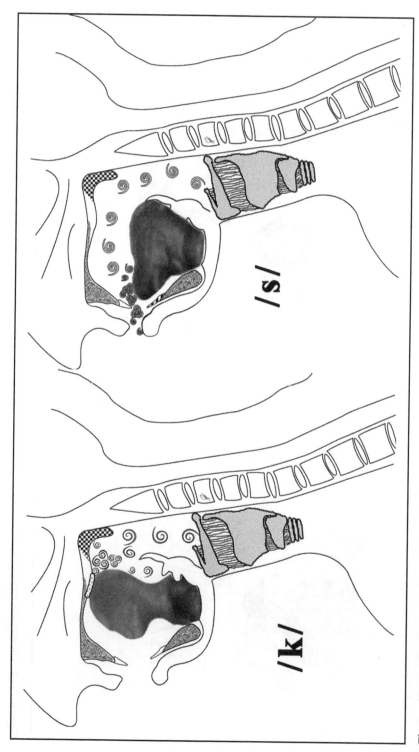

Figure 15–5. Ultrasound representation of /ks/.

Glossary

Abdomen: the large body cavity between the pelvic floor and the diaphragm that contains the abdominal viscera.

Abdominal: pertaining to the abdomen.

Abduction: the movement of *vocal folds* away from their centerline due to the force of pressurized air moving up through the vocal folds.

Ach-laut: /ɑχlaᵘt/, a *phoneme* found in both German and Hebrew that is produced with high *subglottal* pressure in which the back of the tongue interacts with the *soft palate*. (This phoneme has no equivalent in English.) It is employed after the written vowels a, o, u, or the diphthong au. (Examples include Nacht /naχt/; hoch /hɔχ/; and lachen /lʌχən/.

Acoustic singing: singing that is not electronically amplified in a large space such as a concert hall.

Acoustical reflector: distribute and reflect sound.

Adduct: the movement of the *vocal folds* toward the centerline due to a combination of *myoelasticity* and the *Bernoulli effect*. See also *Abduction*.

Adduction: see *Adduct*.

Affricate: a compound *consonant* that begins as a *stop* and is released as a *fricative* (i.e., /dʒ/).

Airway: a tube-like anatomical structure that conveys air from the atmosphere and the lungs during *respiration*.

Alveolar ridge: /ælviɔlɚ/, the ridge of the gum behind the upper teeth.

Alveopalatals: see *Alveolar ridge* and Palatal.

Amplitude: the degree of displacement of a vibrating object. The greater the distance the object moves from its centerline during vibration, the greater is the amplitude. Our perception of loudness is partially derived from the degree of amplitude.

Amplitude versus time: referring to *spectrograms*; time is represented on the *x*-axis, left to right, and amplitude on the *y*-axis, bottom to top.

Anatomy: the study of the physical structure of the human body.

Antagonism: the opposition of force supplied by two opposing muscles. The ratio of the opposition determines the force exerted in a given direction.

Angle (of the mandible/jaw): where the body and ramus connect.

Antagonists: muscles of opposition; those muscles that counter the force of another so that the ratio of forces between them allows very fine control over muscular force.

Anterior: toward the front of a structure (opposite of *posterior*).

Aperiodic: /eⁱpɪriɑdɪk/, *vibrations* that occur at irregular *periods*.

Aperture: degree of opening.

Articular disc: a thin, oval plate of fibrocartilage present in several joints to allow for movement.

Articulate: to utilize the *articulators* of the *vocal tract* to create language sounds.

Articulators: structures in the *vocal tract* that can be used singly or interactively to create speech or singing language sounds—that is, tongue, lips, teeth, *soft palate,* and hard palate.

Arytenoid: /ɑrɪtɛnoⁱd/, one of a pair of movable *cartilages* in the *larynx* that serve as posterior attachment points for the *vocal folds.*

Aspirate: /æspərət/, a *consonant* created by bringing the *vocal folds* to the *laryngeal* centerline just slightly outside the *aperture* needed for *phonation* resulting in *turbulence* that is heard as an /h/.

Attenuate: to lessen.

Back vowel: a class of vowel in which the tongue moves back in the mouth and thereby creates a major *resonance* space in the front of the mouth with a corresponding smaller space *posterior* to the tongue.

Belt: the technique of carrying the *chest voice* tone progressively higher past the *primary register transition (PRT).* This production is commonly used by *contemporary commercial music (CCM)* singers in the popular, folk, and musical theater genres.

Benchmark: a standard by which other like things are judged.

Benchmark exercise: An exercise for improving resonance in *consonant-to-vowel (CV)* joins. In the benchmark, the singer utilizes a rich, well-sung vowel to bracket a consonant that is in need of adjustment. The vowel is sung first, followed by the consonant, and then the singer returns to the vowel without

stopping. The presence of the two benchmark vowels helps maximize the *resonance* of the *consonant.* Terms first introduced by Garyth Nair.

Bernoulli effect (principle): named after Daniel Bernoulli (pronounced /bə-nuli/), an 18th-century Swiss mathematician and physician who developed the kinetic theory of fluids. The principle states that at a point of constriction, a stream of fluid (air in the case of the voice) must simultaneously undergo a decrease in pressure and an increase in particle velocity.

Bilabial: two lips. See also *Labia.*

Biofeedback: information that provides external *KR* in the learning process via mechanical or electronic means. See also *Feedback.*

BIVYN: the acronym for the principle, **Breathe In The Vowel You Need.** Also referred to by the icon. Terms first introduced by Garyth Nair.

Blade (of the tongue): the top front surface of the tongue, also called the *dorsum.*

Body (of the mandible/jaw): the curved, somewhat horseshoe-like shape holding the lower teeth in place

Bolus: /bəᵘləs/, a round mass, specifically a soft mass of chewed food in the mouth or esophagus.

Boyle's law: in an enclosed container holding an amount of fluid (gas or liquid), an increase in the size (volume) of the container will lower the pressure of the fluid. Applied to the voice, an increase in the volume of the lungs will result in a decrease of the air pressure and will result in the influx of more air in order to equalize that pressure (inhalation).

Break: a transition point between vocal *registers.* See also *Primary register transition, Lift,* and *Passaggio.*

Broadband display: type of spectro-graphic display where the bandwidth is set wide. In this analysis, individual harmonics are difficult to identify but formant frequencies are easier. This display is sometimes very useful in cases of vowel identity or vowel drift problems.

Bühnenaussprache: /bʏnənaᵘsʃpraçə/, stage diction. A dialect-less version of the German language used in German theaters.

Call: a register violation that occurs above the *primary register transition (PRT)* that sounds very forced and strained, often produced with extreme tensing of laryngeal muscles. Also referred to as the "shout."

Cartilage: /kartəlædʒ/, a firm and flex-ible connective tissue; particularly prominent in the larynx and respiratory system.

Caudal: toward the bottom of the body.

CCM: see *Contemporary commercial music.*

Centering: keeping the vocal production on the imaginary centerline that runs up through the abdomen, chest, neck, and out through the mouth. Remem-bering to center one's vocal production adds greatly in preventing *spreading.*

Central vowel: a vowel produced with the tongue at or near the rest or neutral position.

Chest voice: the lower of the two *primary registers* in the human voice. It is produced with much more vocal fold mass than its corollary, the *head voice.*

Clavicles: /klævəkəlz/, two bones in the skeletal complex of the shoulders. The clavicles are the prominent bow-shaped bones on the front of the shoulder leading to the centerline of the chest.

Coarticulation: a state where the produc-tion of one *phoneme* influences the production of the *phonemes* on either side of it; this can result in a distur-bance in the clarity and/or *timbre* of the surrounding sounds.

Complex periodic vibration: a sound that regularly repeats a pattern of simul-taneously sounding, mathematically predictable *partials.*

Concomitant: occurring at the same time.

Condyle: /kɒndʌɪl/, the round promi-nence at the end of a bone, most often part of a joint—an articulation with another bone, such as the *temporoman-dibular joint (TMJ).*

Consonant: one of the two principal classes of language sounds, *vowels* and *consonants.* Consonants are those *phonemes* that are not *vowels* and are executed with a partial or complete constriction of the *vocal tract.*

Consonant resonance: A term and concept first introduced by Garyth Nair. Concept of maintaining a vowel-like *resonance* behind the point of constriction or *occlusion* that is needed in the production of *consonants.* Also referred to in this text by its acronym, *CR.*

Consonant shadow: a term used in the author's studio for any form of *coarticulation* caused by the presence of a consonant. Just like a shadow cast by light, the poorly performed consonant can cast an acoustic shadow on the phoneme on either side of it. Terms first introduced by Garyth Nair.

Consovowel: consonants that have a pitch component (such as /z/, /ʒ/, /m/, /n/, and /ŋ/) that can be sung with a vowel-like resonance.

Consovowel practice: a technique of singing a text articulating only vowels and *consovowels* so as to equalize *reso-nance* in the line.

Constriction: to contract or shrink (as opposed to occlude, close, or shut a passage).

Contemporary commercial music (CCM): a term used to denote nonclassical singing.

Continuants: vocal sounds that can be sustained because the airflow in the *vocal tract* is not totally blocked. The sound can be sustained for as long as *subglottal pressure* can be maintained on one breath.

Coronoid process: /kɔrɔnoⁱd/ (from Greek *korone*, "like a crown"), is a thin, triangular eminence (elevation) on the jawbone.

CR: see *Consonant resonance.*

Cranial: toward the skull of the body.

Cricoarytenoid: /krʌiko arɪtɛnoⁱd/, two muscles that open and close the glottis. The lateral cricoarytenoid closes the space and the posterior cricoarytenoid opens it. The two muscles work as antagonists to create the precise glottal aperture necessary for phonation.

Cricothyroid (CT): /krʌiko θʌⁱrɔⁱd/, the *vocal fold* lengthening muscles. When these muscles contract, the *thyroid cartilage* is pulled down and forward toward the *cricoid* cartilage. Also known as lengthener muscles.

CV: a *consonant-to-vowel join.* Example: the syllable "me" in the word "memory" features a shift from the consonant /m/ to the vowel /ɛ/. See also *VC.*

Cycle: one complete set of regularly recurring actions. Generally used to describe cycles in time (cps, cycles per second, or *Hz*). Used in conjunction with descriptions of *vibratory* properties.

dB: abbreviation for *decibel.*

Decibel: /dɛsəbəl/, a logarithmic measurement of sound pressure named to honor Alexander Graham Bell's pioneering work with vocal acoustics.

Depress: push or pull something down into a lower position.

Diacritic (diacritical): any mark(s) set around a printed letter or phonetic symbol that alter its pronunciation, such as the two dots present over one of three German vowels, ü, ö, and ä. See also *Umlaut.*

Dialect: a variety of spoken language produced by geographic, political, social, or economic isolation.

Diphthong: /dɪfθɑŋ/, two consecutive *vowels* occurring in the same syllable with one vowel getting the lion's share of the production time. In this book, we refer to the sustained vowel as the *primary* and the short tag-vowel as *secondary.* The secondary vowel can either precede or follow the primary. Examples would be the English word "may," in which the /e/ is sustained far longer than the /i/ that completes the diphthong (/meⁱ/). A *secondary*-initial diphthong is the word "yes" /ʲɛs/. Also note that in this book, we always superscript the *secondary* vowel in *IPA* transliterations.

Dorsum: see *Blade (of the tongue).*

Dynamic: pertaining to musical notation that indicates loudness such as *p, f,* and *mf.*

Dysphonia: /dɪsfoniʌ/, impairment of voicing (*phonation*).

Elastic: see *Elasticity.*

Elasticity: the property of a substance that causes it to return to its original shape after having been deformed.

Electromyograph: (abbreviated *EMG*) an instrument that reads electrical activity in muscles. The electromyography employed in voice research is one that is invasive—that is, tiny electrodes are placed in the muscle to be studied.

Another type of electromyography is the surface electromyograph, an instrument that reads muscle tension by way of sensitive pads placed on the skin over the muscles in question. Due to the number of artifacts generally produced in this type of electromyography, it is not used in research but may be utilized as an adjunct in biofeedback applications.

Electromyography: the use of the *electromyograph.*

Electropalatography: (abbreviated *EPG*) a technique used to monitor contacts between the tongue and hard palate, particularly during articulation and speech.

EMG: see *Electromyograph.*

Endorphins: natural "feel good" hormones originating in our brains that can elevate our mood.

Envisioning: using one's imagination to "see" one's self-executing or performing a certain task. This technique helps one plan all the nonmusical/nonartistic things that must happen during a performance.

EPG: see *Electropalatography.*

Epiglottis: /ɛpɪɡlɑtəs/, the *cartilage* flap that seals the top of the *larynx* during swallowing.

Epilaryngeal tube: /ɛpɪlɑrɪndʒʲəl/, the small *resonator* in the vocal tract bound by the *glottis* (the closed end) and the rim of the epiglottis (the open end that connects to the *pharynx*). The epilaryngeal tube is important to singers because it is thought to be the source of the *singer's formant.*

Epilarynx: /ɛpɪlærɪŋks/, a small resonating region bound by the rim of the *epiglottis* and the *glottis.* This is the area where the *singer's formant* is thought to originate. The term *epilaryngeal tube* is synonymous with epilarynx.

Equilibrium stance: a way of standing with one foot slightly ahead of the other. This stance permits a wider circle of balance than any other way of positioning one's feet.

Exhale: pushing air out of the lungs and *airway* during the act of *respiration.*

Exit: 1. The act of ceasing *phonation.* 2. The act of leaving the stage.

Extrinsic: outside of.

f_0: scientific shorthand for the *fundamental* (if you think of this as standing for *frequency of oscillation*, it will be easy to remember). Note, in most sources this term is shown as F_0. In this text, the series of various overtones are listed $1f_o$, $2f_o$, $3f_o$, etc.

Fascia: a band or sheet of connective tissue that connects muscles to other muscles.

F-pattern: *formant* pattern. The relative placement of the formants on the sound spectrum. Each vowel has its own predictable F-pattern.

Feedback: modification or control of a process or system by its results or effects. This is different from *biofeedback*, where an external stimulus is used to acquire voluntary control of a process or system.

Fluid: a nonsolid substance such as a liquid or a gas that tends to conform to the shape of its container.

Forced resonator: the *resonator* of a musical instrument that sympathetically takes the sound of the *tone generator* and amplifies it. Example: the soundboard of a piano.

Formant: a vocal-tract resonance. It appears on *spectrograms* as a bright cluster of prominent *harmonics.* Formants alter the source signal emanating from the *vocal folds* and permit us to produce our various *vowels* and can also influence the sound of the *consovowels*.

Formant tuning: manipulation (retuning) of principally the f_1 (first *formant*) frequency by physical means to maintain an acoustic coupling with f_O as a means of avoiding register violations.

Frontal (coronal): dividing the body into front and back (anterior and posterior or ventral and dorsal)

Frequency: the rate of repetition of a *periodic* event. In sound, it is the number of vibrational *cycles* per second and is expressed in *hertz (Hz)*. This word is not equivalent to the word *pitch,* which is a human perception of *frequency.*

Frequency versus amplitude: the graphical display of a *power spectrum* where *frequency* is represented on the horizontal axis and *amplitude* on the vertical axis.

Fricative: /frɪkətɪv/, a *consonant* produced by constricting the *vocal tract* to produce pitchless *turbulence* (i.e., /f/, /v/, /s/, etc.).

Front vowel: a *vowel* that requires the tongue to shift forward of its at-rest (neutral) position. This creates a small *resonance* in the front of the mouth and a large one at the back. Examples are /i/, /e/, /ɪ/, and so forth.

Fundamental: the lowest harmonic of a periodic waveform, written as f_O.

Genio-: /dʒɛnio/, prefix for "chin."

Genioglossus: /dʒɛnioɡlɑsəs/, the prime articulator of the tongue that radiates from the chin (*genio*) and inserts in the tongue (*glossus*); it also inserts into the *hyoid bone* (as such, it can elevate the *hyoid* and, hence, the *larynx*).

Geniohyoid: /dʒɛniohʌˈɔˈd/, a muscle that inserts into the *hyoid bone* and connects to the *mandible*. Like the *genioglossus,* it can elevate the hyoid bone, or if that bone is fixed, it can lower the mandible.

Gesamtkunstwerk: total work of art.

Glide: a written *consonant* that is actually a vowel sound, produced in transition to a following *vowel* (e.g., /ʷ/ or /ʲ/).

Glossus: /ɡlɑsəs/, the tongue.

Glottal: /ɡlɑtəl/, pertaining to the *glottis.*

Glottal closing: the motion of the vocal folds toward the centerline of the larynx.

Glottal opening: the motion of the vocal folds away from the centerline of the larynx.

Glottal stop: the precipitous and plosive release of air pressure that has been built below a full *occlusion* of the vocal folds. If performed chronically and with sufficient force, the use of glottal stops can contribute to vocal fold injury.

Glottal stroke: a transient *glottal* event where the vocal folds remain closed for a slightly longer time than the normal *Close Quotion* time. This allows for a slight buildup of air pressure that is released as a gentle *plosive*. It is commonly used in language to separate *phonemes* where meaning of words might be misconstrued, for example, "some ice" being heard as "some mice" if no glottal stroke intercedes between the /m/ of "some" and the /aⁱ/ of "ice."

Glottis: /ɡlɑtəs/, the space between the *vocal folds.*

GRAM: a freeware spectrographic program, written by Richard Horne, that is used in the examples throughout this text. More professional variants of the program are available from Horne at https://www.visualizationsoftware. com/gram. Other software is also available at https://www.sygyt.com/en/.

Habituate: to cause an action to become habit.

Hard r: see *Retroflex* /ɹ/.

Harmonic amplitude: the loudness of a give *harmonic* in a musical *tone.*

Harmonics: mathematically predictable *vibrations*, higher in frequency and less in amplitude than the *fundamental* (f_o) simultaneously occurring in a vibration. Thus, its various overtones are listed as $1f_o$, $2f_o$, $3f_o$, etc.). Note, in this book we adapt the old notations of harmonics (H_1, H_2, H_3, etc.) with the new one. Such harmonics are a function of the fundamental, and differences in their *amplitude* are responsible for the character of the sound we hear (*timbre*).

Head voice: one of the two principal modes of *vibration* produced by the *vocal folds*. In head voice, the mass of the folds is much less than in *chest voice*, and *phonation* is mostly accomplished by the edge of the vocal fold *mucosa*.

Hertz: /hɝts/, one complete cycle of a periodic vibration. Named for the physicist, Heinrich Hertz. See also *Frequency* and *Hz*.

Hochdeutsch: /hɔχdɔⁱtʃ/, "high German," a *dialect*-less version of the German language. Hochdeutsch is commonly used by professional singers and other professional users of the voice such as actors and broadcasters. See also *Bühnenaussprache*.

Hyoglossus: /hʌⁱoglɑsʊs/, a laterally placed muscle with the origin in the upper side of the *hyoid bone* that inserts into the tongue.

Hyoid bone: /hʌⁱɔⁱd/, a U-shaped bone below the base of the tongue that connects both the tongue and the *larynx* by means of *ligaments*.

Hz: abbreviation for *hertz*.

Ich-laut: /içlaᵘt/, a German *fricative phoneme* formed by a semioccluding high arch of the tongue that modifies the *PoA (Place of Articulation)* of the English /k/. A small opening is allowed at the center of the tongue arch that creates the *turbulence* associated with the proper performance of this phoneme. German abounds with Ich-lauts (e.g., *icht* as in *nicht*—/nıçt/).

Inferior: below.

Inhalation: the act of drawing in air during respiration. See also *Inspiration*.

Inspiration: synonym for *inhalation*, the act of drawing in air during *respiration*.

Intercostal: external and internal muscles between the ribs that are involved in the process of inhalation/exhalation.

International Phonetic Alphabet: (abbreviated *IPA*) a notational system in which each symbol represents a *phoneme*, an individual acoustic block of language

Interoral pressure: (abbreviated P_{io}) air pressure in the oral and *pharyngeal* cavities *superior* to the *glottis*.

Intrinsic: inside.

IPA: see *International Phonetic Alphabet*; it can also refer to the International Phonetic Association.

Jaw: the bone that hinges downward from the *TMJ* and houses the teeth and the tongue.

Join: the point of change between two sequential *phonemes*.

Labial: /leⁱbiəl/, pertaining to the lips. See also *Labio-*.

Labio-: pertaining to the lips. See also *Labial*.

Labiodental: a *consonant* produced with the lower lip contacting the bottom of the upper front teeth.

Laryngeal: /lɑrındʒəl/, pertaining to the larynx.

Larynges: /lɑrındʒiz/, plural of *larynx*.

Larynx: the vocal organ situated in the neck that houses the *vocal folds*. Pronounced /larıŋks/, not /larniks/.

Lateral: away from the center on the horizontal plane, toward the outside.

Laut-: /laᵘt/, German word for "sound." Used in conjunction with *Ich-* and

Ach- to describe specific German *frica-tive* phonemes, the *Ich-laut* (/ç/) and the *Ach-laut* (/χ/).

Lied: /liːt/ (plural *Lieder* /lidɚ/), German art songs based on Germanic poetry of the Romantic era. Lieder music was written primarily for the enjoyment of amateur musicians in their homes.

Lieder: the plural of the German word, *Lied.*

Lift: a transition point between vocal *registers.* See also *Break* and *Passaggio.*

Ligament: strong tissue that connects bones and holds organs in place.

Lingua: referring to the tongue. See also *Lingual.*

Linguadental: a *consonant* produced with tongue-teeth contact.

Lingual: referring to the tongue. See also *Lingua.*

Linguapalatal: a *consonant* produced with tongue-hard palate contact. Also called *Palatal.*

Liquids: *consovowels* made with an incomplete *occlusion* between the tongue and the roof of the mouth (such as the consovowel /l-/).

LMM: see *Low mandible maneuver.*

Loft voice: another term for the vocal *register* above the middle voice. Sometimes also called *falsetto* in scientific literature.

Longitudinal movement: movement of the tongue on its *anterior/posterior* axis (front to back). In speech, this movement is called tongue advancement.

Loudness: the perceived strength of a sound (as opposed to its measurable *amplitude* which is not necessarily the same value).

Low mandible maneuver: (abbreviated *LMM*) the drop of the posterior (back) mandible (jaw), increasing oral (mouth) and pharyngeal (behind the mouth and above the larynx) cavity.

Lungs: the structures we use to momentarily store inhaled air during the reparatory cycle. The exchange of blood gases, oxygen for carbon dioxide occurs in the lungs.

Mandible: the jawbone including the *ramus.*

Mandible elevation: the relative position of the *mandible* on the vertical plane.

Medial: meaning toward the center (midplane or midline). *Mesial* is a synonym for medial.

Melisma: two or more notes sung on a single syllable.

Messa: Italian for "putting" or "placing," used in the term for the classic Italian exercise, *messa di voce.*

Messa di voce: performance of a long crescendo from piano to forte and then, just as evenly, a diminuendo back to piano. *Messa di voce* is the classical volume-control exercise.

Millisecond: (abbreviated *ms* or *msec*) one-thousandth of a second.

ms: abbreviation for *millisecond* or one-thousandth of a second.

msec: abbreviation for *millisecond* or one-thousandth of a second.

Muscle memory: the ability to move a muscle system to a relatively specific point in space. The memory is acquired after many successful repetitions of the movement.

Muscular hydrostat: muscular organ that lacks typical systems of skeletal support; the most important biomechanical feature is that its volume is constant.

Musical tone: a mathematically predictable sequence of *harmonics*; the opposite of *noise.*

Myo-: /mʌⁱoᵘ/, pertaining to muscle tissue.

Myoelasticity: muscle *elasticity*; the tendency of a muscle to return to its place of rest after being moved, stretched, or tightened.

Narrowband display: a type of spectrographic display that uses a narrow bandwidth. In this analysis image, individual *harmonics* are visible as narrow bands streaming across the screen. *Formants* can be seen as areas of darkness surrounding the appropriate harmonics. For most voice *feedback* work, this is the preferred bandwidth because so many acoustic details are clearly represented. For formant identity, the narrowband display is not as useful as the *broadband display*.

Nasal: pertaining to the nose.

Nasopharynx: /neizofæriŋks/, the area of the *pharynx* leading from the *nasal* passages down to the *oropharynx*.

Neuromuscular abilities: the interplay between the brain (command) and a muscle (task).

Neutral vowel: a vowel made in the center of the *oral* cavity. Two neutral *phonemes*, the schwa, /ə/ and /ʌ/ (as well as the *rhoticized schwas*) are made in that region. See also *Front* and *Back Vowels*.

Noise: the lack of cyclically reoccurring patterns of complex *vibration* (i.e., no ordered structure of *harmonics* over the f_0).

Obstruent: a speech sound formed by obstructing airflow.

Occlusion: complete closure of a passageway.

Offglide: term used by phoneticians for the transition from a *vowel* of longer duration to one of shorter duration (e.g., /ʌⁱ/, as in the word "eye"). See also *Primary vowel, Secondary vowel,* and *Glide*.

Offset: how a singer ends a *vowel phoneme* when going into silence; the opposite of *onset*.

Onglide: term used by phoneticians for the transition from a *vowel* of shorter duration to one of longer duration (e.g., /ʲu/, as in the word "you"). See also *Primary vowel, Secondary vowel,* and *Glide*.

Onset: the act of initiating *phonation* following silence.

Oral: pertaining to the mouth.

Oral cavity: the space within the mouth.

Oropharynx: the area of the pharynx posterior (behind) to the oral cavity.

Oscillation: a back-and-forth movement that is repeated.

Overtone: a component of the sound spectrum that is an integer multiple of the *fundamental* (f_0). Overtones are numbered beginning with the first component above the fundamental (hence the part of the word, "over"). Not to be confused with the terms *partial* or *harmonic* that include the fundamental as part of the numbered series.

Palatal: 1. A *consonant* produced with tongue-hard palate contact. Also called *linguapalatal*. 2. Pertaining to the palate, the roof of the mouth.

Palate: the roof of the mouth that includes both the hard palate (*anterior* or *front*) and the *soft palate* or *velum* (*posterior* or *back*).

Palatogram: a graphic representation of the degree of tongue-molar contact as viewed from below the jaw.

Para-affricate: term for consonant combinations that begin as a *stop plosive* and end with a release similar to another consonant. In linguistics, only the /dʒ/ is considered an *affricate*. However, there are other *phonemes* that begin as a stop plosive and are released as another consonant, such as the phoneme /ts/. In this text, we refer to these phonemes as para-affricates. Term first introduced by Garyth Nair.

Partial: a component of the sound spectrum that is an integer multiple of the *fundamental* (f_o). Unlike the related terms *overtone* and *harmonics*, the numbering of the partials includes the fundamental in the series (i.e., the first harmonic is also called the first partial). See also *Overtone* and *Harmonic*.

Passaggio: /pasadʒɔ/ (plural, *passaggi*, / pasasdʒi/) 1. The point of shift between two vocal *registers*. This is the preferred definition in the voice science literature. 2. The area (usually four notes) surrounding the shift point between registers where the singer must gradually move the mode of vocal production from one register to the other. This definition is usually employed by teachers and teachers of singing. Technically, this area should be called the *zona di passaggio*.

Pedagogy: a teaching philosophy or method.

Pelvic: pertaining to the pelvis.

Period: an action or collection of actions that regularly, and thus predictably, reoccurs.

Periodic: a regularly recurring action or set of actions.

Perturbation: /pɝtɝbeiʃən/, minor changes from expected behavior.

Pharynx: /færɪŋks/, the airway of the upper respiratory system from *velum* to the top of the *larynx*.

Phonation: vibration of the vocal folds during the production of vowels or pitch consonants. (There is also a brief moment of *phonation* during the *prevoicing* of the *prevoiced* pitch *consonants* such as /b/ or /d/.)

Phoneme: a unique unit of sound within a specific language.

Phonemic: pertaining to *phonemes*.

Phonetician: one who deals with phonetics

Phonetics: the study and classification of speech sounds

Physics: the study of the physical forces (mechanics) of nature.

Physioacoustics: a term introduced by Garyth Nair for the study of the relationship between the *anatomy* and *physiology* of the singing voice and the radiated result.

Physiology: the study of the function of how the parts of the body work, both individually and in concert with each other.

Pitch: a listener's perception of the highness or lowness of a tone, based on *frequency*.

Plosive: a synonym for *stop consonants*; sometimes also called *stop-plosives*.

Place of articulation: (abbreviated *PoA*) *consovowels* and *consonants* are produced by executing an *occlusion* or *constriction* at a specific place in the *oral cavity*. The point of articulation is the place at which the occlusion/constriction is produced.

PoA: see *Place of articulation*.

Posterior: toward the back of a structure.

Power spectrum: a type of sound analysis that produces a two-dimensional graphic in which the *x*-axis shows *frequency* and the *y*-axis shows *amplitude*. The power spectrum displays the analysis of sound at a given point in time (the opposite of the *spectrogram* that shows a scrolling display along the *x*-axis that denotes the passage of time).

Pressed voice: *phonation* produced by a tight *glottal* focus and high *subglottal* pressure. It is a mode of *phonation* that is considered as voice abuse and can lead to nodules.

Prevoiced stop: a stop *consonant* that is preceded by a *prevoicing*. See also *Simple stop*.

Prevoicing: momentary occluded *phonation* that occurs prior to the release of pressure in a *prevoiced* stop. The prevoicing is performed with the vocal instrument sealed so the time that the momentary *phonation* can occur is as brief as the time required to equalize the *subglottal* and *supraglottal* pressure. At that point in time, the built-up pressure is released as a stop *consonant*. Because the prevoicing is sung on a *pitch,* the pitch permeates through the release of the pressure component.

Primary and secondary vowels: terminology for the two monophthongs of a *diphthong* (first introduced by Garyth Nair). In singing, the primary vowel is sustained for a longer period of time than its corollary in a spoken diphthong. The *secondary vowel* is the monophthong that takes minimal execution time in a sung diphthong. These terms, suggested by the author, are meant to replace the speech terms, *onglide, offglide,* and nucleus, when discussing sung diphthongs. In this text, the *secondary vowel* of the diphthong is indicated by superscripting (i.e., /ɑⁱ/ as in the word "my").

Primary register: the two basic *vibratory* modes that our *vocal folds* can produce: the *chest voice* (or heavy *vibratory* mode) occurring below the *primary register transition* and the *head voice* (or lighter *vibratory* mode)—the notes of the scale above the primary register transition.

Primary register transition: (abbreviated *PRT*) the point in a sung scale at which the *larynx* naturally wants to shift from one *primary register* to the other.

Proprioceptor: specialized type of neuron that among other information, allows us to know where parts of our body are in space. This information is based on the neurons reading the relative amount of muscle stretching occurring.

Protrusion: an extension beyond the normal line or surface.

PRT: see *Primary register transition.*

P_sub: see *Subglottal pressure.*

Radiated signal: the completed vocal sound, the combination of the *source signal* and the *supraglottal resonances* that leave the mouth of the singer.

Ramus: the vertical, *posterior* part of the jaw that *articulates* with the skull.

Range: 1. The compass between the lowest and highest written notes in a song. 2. All the notes from the bottom to the top of an individual voice.

Rate: term applied to *vibrato* indicating the number of vibrato *cycles* per second.

Real time: a result that appears virtually simultaneous with its cause. A *spectrogram* is said to be running in *virtual real time* when the lag between the sound produced by the subject and its appearance on the monitor is short enough that the subject does not consciously sense the lag.

Register: an area of the voice where the *timbre* of the voice remains basically the same for a contiguous portion of the singer's *range.*

Register transition: the method by which a singer moves from one vocal *register* to another.

Register tuning: the theory of vocal *register transition* that concentrates on physical manipulation of the *vocal folds* to impart or subtract mass.

Resonance: the sympathetic *vibratory* response to *sound* waves.

Resonator: 1. A physical entity that is set into *vibration* by the proximity of another *vibration.* In the human voice, the resonator consists of all the air-filled *supraglottal* spaces. 2. An object or space that has *resonance.*

Respiration: the act of breathing in and out; *inhalation/exhalation.*

Respiratory: pertaining to the act of *respiration*, breathing.

Retroflex: /ɹ/, a *phoneme* that is commonly called the *hard r*. It is produced by pulling the tip of the tongue back in the oral cavity from the more neutral r-position. As the tongue is pulled back, it creates a highly concave tongue shape that creates a very brittle, *spread* sound.

Rhotic: /roᵘtɪk/; rhoticized: a *vowel* sound produced with r-coloring.

Rhoticized schwa: a *schwa* /ə/ produced with a slight /r/ color and commonly called a *schwar*. The *IPA* symbol for the schwar is /ɚ/.

Sagittal: /sædʒətəl/, an imaginary slice down the center of the anatomy as viewed from the side.

SAS: /sæs/, acronym adopted by Garyth Nair for "say it as a singer," an exercise where a singer/actor speaks the words of a song with full singer's resonance. The exercise helps the student with the idea of the radical shift from the speech over to the singing template.

Scapula: shoulder blade or wing bone.

Schwa: /ʃʷɑ/, the schwa is a neutral vowel (indicated by the *IPA* symbol /ə/) employed exclusively for unaccented syllables in English and German. It also appears in other languages such as French. See also *Rhoticized schwa*.

Schwar: /ʃʷɑr/, the *word-final* unaccented "er" in English and indicated by the *IPA* symbol /ɚ/. Although r is a *consovowel*, the combination of written "e" and "r" is actually a *vowel* in its own right.

Scooping: the conscious or unconscious failure to begin a *vowel* or *consovowel* precisely on pitch. Scoops occur from below the pitch and achieve the pitch or record within a few milliseconds. Within the norms of classical technique, scooping is not a desirable trait in a singer.

Scrolling: the ribbonlike display of a real-time spectrogram.

Secondary vowel: see *Primary vowel* and *Diphthongs*.

Semienclosed airspace: a type of *resonator*. Examples in music include wind and brass instruments, flutelike organ pipes, and the human voice.

Semivowel: a *consonant* that has vowel-like *resonance*. See also *Consovowel*.

Set-energize: A technique developed by Garyth Nair of making sure that all *articulators* are in precise position needed for the first language sound before energy is committed to the *vocal folds* to cause *phonation*.

Sibilants: *unvoiced fricatives* that have more energy in the upper realms of the *spectrum* such as /s/, /dʒ/, and /ʃ/, and the *consovowel* /ʒ/.

Simple harmonic motion: smoothest possible back-and-forth motion.

Simple stop: *stop* consonants that have no *pitch* element (i.e., /t/, /k/, and /p/). See also *Prevoiced stop*.

Singer's formant: an area of vocal *resonance* in the area between 2.3 and 3.5 kHz that singers call "ring" or "point." It imparts brilliance to the voice that is principally associated with Western concert and operatic singing styles.

Sinus: a semienclosed area in the body containing air (as in the maxillary sinuses, or the piriform sinuses).

Soft palate: the *velum*, the *posterior* roof of the mouth that is made up of *palatal* muscles covered with a *mucosal* membrane.

Sound: the product of a vibrating object in which the energy created by movement of the *oscillating* material travels through a medium such as air.

Sound pressure level: (abbreviated *SPL*) the measurable pressure sound waves exert on the eardrum.

Source filter theory: a theory developed by Gunnar Fant, later expanded by Johan Sundberg (and others) in which *vocal tract resonances* (*formants*) alter the *harmonic amplitude* of the *source signal* from the *vocal folds*. This manipulation results in the almost infinite variety of radiated *timbre* that comprise language and vocal *tone*.

Source signal: the sound originating from the *vocal folds* before any *resonance* effect is applied by the *supraglottal* resonances.

Spectrogram: a three-dimensional computer-generated graphic representation of the analysis of sound showing time on the horizontal axis, *frequency* on the vertical axis, and *amplitude* as intensity of color or grayscale. If the *spectrogram* is running in *real time*, it is said to be *scrolling*.

Spectrograph: the apparatus or computer software that produces a *spectrogram*.

Spectrum: an array of entities ordered by magnitude. In sound spectrography, there are two basic types of spectra (pl.), the *spectrogram* and the *power spectrum*.

Speech-based: the phonemes of the language being sung are produced in almost the same manner as when the singer is speaking

Spike: the thin vertical component of the spectrographic display that results from the performance of a *transient* (such as the *consonant* /t/).

Spine: the vertical column of bones that runs from the base of the *pelvis* to the skull. See also *Vertebrae*.

SPL: see *Sound pressure level*.

Spreading: the use of oral-facial musculature that directs air and sound out through a narrow horizontal opening rather than a vertical plane.

Sternum: commonly called the breastbone, the sternum is the connection point for the seven true ribs and three false ribs.

Stop or **stop consonant:** a *consonant* produced by building air pressure behind an *occlusion* of the vocal cavity and then suddenly releasing that pressure. See also *Simple stop* and *Prevoiced stop*. (Also known as a *plosive*.)

Stop plosive: see *Stop consonant*.

Subglottal: airways below the *glottis*.

Subglottal pressure: (abbreviated P_{sub}) muscularly produced air pressure below the *glottis*.

Suboccipital muscles: short neck muscles; a group of four muscles situated underneath the occipital bone (bone which forms the back and base of the skull).

Superior: above.

Support: the controlled delivery of pressurized *subglottal* airflow to the *vocal folds* during singing. It is achieved by the *abdominal* muscles exerting inward and upward pressure on the abdominal *viscera* (contents of the abdominal cavity which include the large and small intestines, the stomach, the liver, and so forth) and is controlled by the simultaneous antagonistic action of the *diaphragm* (the muscle of antagonism).

Supra: /suprʌ/, above.

Supraglottal: the *vocal tract* structures above the *glottis*.

Supralaryngeal: refers to anatomical structures located above the *larynx* (i.e., the *oral cavity* and the *pharynx*).

Sustained oscillation: a *vibration* that is sustained by the continuation of the application of energy.

TA: see *Thyroarytenoid*.

Temporomandibular joint: (abbreviated *TMJ*) /tɛmporo mændɪbʲulɚ/, the universal joint between the *ramus* of the *mandible* (jaw) and the skull.

Tendon: a tough band of fibrous connective tissue that connects muscle to the bone.

Tensegrity: coined by the architect R. Buckminster Fuller, is an elision of "tension + integrity," to indicate that the integrity of the structure derived from the balance of tension members, not the compression struts. Tom Myers adapted this concept to the body, particularly the myofascia.

Tessitura: /tɛsitʊrʌ/, the mean pitch area of all the notated pitches to be sung in a work.

Thyroarytenoid: (abbreviated *TA*) /θʌˈroᵘarɪtənɔⁱd/, the muscular core of each vocal fold. It is actually two muscles, the thyromuscularis and the thyrovocalis, that work in tandem. When we refer to the thyrovocalis, we generally abbreviate its name to *vocalis* muscle.

Timbral: /təmbrəl/, pertaining to *timbre*.

Timbre: /tæmbɚ/, the unique quality of a sound as determined by the relative *amplitude* of its *harmonics,* those acoustic markers that make a sound unique. We speak of the timbre of an oboe versus that of a clarinet. The word *timbre* is not a judgment of quality (that oboe does not sound good) but describes its "oboe-ness."

TMJ: see *Temporomandibular joint.*

Tone: 1. The acoustic characteristics of a musical sound. See also *Timbre.* 2. A pitch sounded by a musical instrument.

Tone generator: a vibrating object that produces sound. In the human voice, the tone generator is the *larynx,* specifically the pair of *vocal folds* found within that organ.

Transducer: a device that converts energy from one form to another. Crystals in the transducer emanate ultra-high-frequency sound waves and produce an image by using their reflective properties, showing the tongue surface and hard palate in real time.

Transient: in linguistics, a brief nonperiodic vocal event such as a /t/. On a spectrogram, transients appear as brief noise spikes on the display.

Transitional belt: the middle voice belt technique that is not a full chest voice production but is attained by physio-acoustic means. See also *Belt.* Term first introduced by Garyth Nair.

Translate: 1. To render the meaning of a foreign language text into another language (usually one's own). 2. To move from one place or condition to another.

Transliterate: to represent the sounds of a language by a system of symbols different from those employed in the everyday written language. *IPA* is the preferred method of transliterating language sounds in the singing repertoire. It has the advantage of representing the actual sounds to be produced rather than the often misleading printed ones. Example: the English word "noise" is transliterated in *IPA* as /noⁱz/. Transliteration can also be called phonetic transcription.

Transliteration: a text that has been *transliterated.*

Transverse: dividing the body into head and tail (cranial and caudal)

Triphthong: /trifθɑŋ/, three consecutive vowels sounding within one syllable.

Turbulence: when speaking of airflow, the opposite of laminar. Airflow that is *turbulent* contains eddies or *vortices* that can produce noise. Entire classes of *consonants* and some *consovowels* depend on induced turbulence as their origin.

Turbulent: the state of *turbulence*, a chaotic flow of a *fluid*, the opposite of laminar.

Ultrasound: Ultrasound is sound waves with frequencies higher than the upper audible limit of human hearing (from 20 kHz up; 20,000 hertz). Ultrasound is used in many different fields, particularly in medicine, to detect objects and measure distances. In this text, the ultrasound is introduced to be used as an invaluable tool for voice research and biofeedback in the voice studio.

Unvoiced: a language sound made without *phonation* (possessing no *pitch*). Synonymous with *voiceless*.

Uvula: /ˈuvʲulʌ/, the cone-shaped lobe of the lower *medial* border of the *velum*.

VC: a *phonemic join* starting with a *vowel* and followed by a *consonant*. Example: the syllable "em" of the word "memory" in which the articulators must shift from the vowel /ɛ/ to the consonant /m/ in the first syllable. *VC* is the opposite of *CV*.

Velopharyngeal port: the region of the *nasopharynx* that forms a passageway from the nasal cavities to the *pharynx*. This area can be closed by the *posterior velum* (*uvula*).

Velum: /ˈviləm/, the *soft palate*. During language production and swallowing, the *posterior* velum closes the *velopharyngeal port*, an action necessary for the production of most *vowels* and *consonants* as well as a critical component of swallowing.

Vertebrae: the *spine*, a collection of 33 interlinked bones called vertebra that are classified into five regions supporting different regions of the body. The breakdown of vertebra per region is as follows:

- Twelve thoracic, in the area of the rib cage (or thorax)
- Three to four coccygeal (fused into one bone, the coccyx), commonly called the tailbone
- Five lumbar, the lower spine to pelvis
- Five sacral (slightly curved section of the pelvis)
- Seven cervical, in the region of the neck

Vibration: the *oscillating* motion of a fluid or elastic solid that radiates sound energy. In humans, the *vocal folds* vibrate to create the sound source used in the creation of language sounds as well as the pitched tones needed for singing.

Vibrato: /vibratɔ/, a 4 to 6 *Hz* quasi-periodic undulation of both *pitch* and *frequency* found in classical vocal technique.

Vibratory: pertaining to *vibration*.

Virtual real time: a spectrographic display that appears on the computer monitor a few milliseconds after the singer has produced the sound. The singer quickly adjusts to the slight delay, and the display feels like real time. Term first introduced by Garyth Nair.

Vocal cords: common, nonscientific synonym for *vocal folds*; *vocal fold* is the preferred usage.

Vocal folds: a paired system of structures consisting of muscle, ligament, and *mucosal* tissue found in the *larynx*. The vocal folds are *tone generators* for the voice, the source of *phonation* for the voice.

Vocal fry: the low *register* below *chest voice*; an *oscillation* of the *vocal folds* that produces *periodic* disturbances in the airstream with perceived temporal gaps. This type of vocalization is not considered within the norms of good Western classical singing but can be used by a skilled practitioner to simulate extreme low notes (especially as employed by Slavic basses). Also called "pulse voice" or "Strohbass."

Vocal tract: all of the air-filled anatomic structures needed for speech/song production. These structures include the trachea, *larynx, pharynx,* oral cavity, and nasal cavity.

Vocalise: /vokəliz/, a pedagogical or warmup exercise involving *vowels,* either singularly or in multiples. Most singers utilize a *vowel vocalise* that employs only one vowel per exercise.

Voce Vista: an advanced spectrographic program that includes the ability to simultaneously show *EMG* signals. A new version of the program can be obtained at https://www.sygyt.com/en/

Voice box: common, nonscientific synonym for *larynx.*

Voice onset time: (abbreviated *VOT*) the interval between the release of a *stop consonant* and the beginning of *phonation* for the following vowel.

Voiced: a language sound made with *phonation* of the *vocal folds* and has *pitch.* See also *Unvoiced* and *Voiceless.*

Voiceless: synonym for *unvoiced* (i.e., a language sound made without *phonation* of the vocal folds).

Vortice: An area of chaotic flow in a moving *fluid,* the opposite of laminar.

VOT: see *Voice onset time.*

Vowel: a nonconsonant *phoneme* that features *phonation* on *pitch* and a definite *articulator* set that produces specific F_1 and F_2 that is identifiable by the listener.

Vowel collapse: in a word-final vowel, the failure to maintain articulator set while

the vowel is ending leading to a degradation of tone and vowel integrity.

Vowel color: another singer's term for the vowel *timbre* or *klang* of a given vowel.

Vowel formant: the first and second formants (F_1 and F_2), clusters of *harmonics* that together register on the auditory cortex to tell a listener what vowel is being produced.

Vowel identity: how a vowel is perceived by a listener—is it the vowel that is intended? Often, a singer internally senses that he or she is singing the correct vowel; however, in terms of radiated sound, it is not accurate enough for the listener. Terms first introduced by Garyth Nair.

Vowel integrity: the maintenance of the *timbre* of a *vowel* for as long as a particular musical passage requires its use. Terms first introduced by Garyth Nair.

Waveform: graphic representation of vibration that plots *amplitude* versus time.

Word-final: a phoneme that occurs at the end of a word.

Word-initial: a phoneme that occurs at the beginning of a word.

Word-interior: a phoneme that occurs in the interior of a word.

Zona di passaggio: /zona di pɑsɑdʒɔ/, the small area of pitches surrounding the shift from one *register* to another in which the singer must gradually modify the production so the shift is not apparent to the listener. Also called the *zona intermedia.* See also *passaggio.*

Further Reading

Beal, J. C. (2014). *English in modern times*. New York, NY: Routledge.

Deme, A. (2014). Intelligibility of sung vowels: The effect of consonantal context and the onset of voicing. *Journal of Voice, 28*(4), 523.e19–523.e25.

Dobson, E. J. (1985). *English pronunciation 1500–1700* (Vol. II). Oxford, UK: Clarendon Press.

Fogerty, D., & Humes, L. E. (2012). The role of vowel and consonant fundamental frequency, envelope, and temporal fine structure cues to the intelligibility of words and sentences. *Journal of the Acoustical Society of America, 131*(2), 1490–1501.

Gottfried, T. L., & Chew, S. L. (1986). Intelligibility of vowels sung by a countertenor. *Journal of the Acoustical Society of America, 79*, 124–130.

Gramming, P., Sundberg, J., Ternström, S., Leanderson, R., & Perkins, W. H. (1987). Relationship between changes in voice pitch and loudness. *STL-Quarterly Progress and Status Report, 28*(1), 39–55.

Gregg, J. W., & Scherer, R. C. (2005). Vowel intelligibility in classical singing. *Journal of Voice, 20*(2), 198–210.

Hollien, H., Mendes-Schwartz, A. P., & Nielsen, K. (2000). Perceptual confusions of high-pitched sung vowels. *Journal of Voice, 14*, 188–197.

Hunter, E. J., & Titze, I. (2010). Variations in intensity, fundamental frequency, and voicing for teachers in occupational versus non-occupational settings. *Journal of Speech, Language, and Hearing Research, 53*(4), 862–875.

Lee, S.-H., Kwon, H.-J., Choi, H-J., Lee, N-H., Lee S-J., & Jin, S-M. (2008). The singer's formant and speaker's ring resonance: A long-term average spectrum analysis. *Clinical and Experimental Otorhinolaryngology, 1*(2), 92–96.

Marshall, M. (1953). *The singer's manual of English diction*. New York, NY: Schirmer.

Miller, G. A., & Nicely, P. E. (1955). An analysis of perceptual confusions among some English consonants. *Journal of the Acoustical Society of America, 27*, 338–353.

Öhman, S. E. G. (1966). Coarticulation in VCV utterances: Spectrographic measurements. *Journal of the Acoustical Society of America, 39*, 151–168.

Rodet, X. (2008). Methods for singing voice control and synthesis. *Journal of the Acoustical Society of America, 123*, 3378.

Strang, B. M. H. (2015). *A history of English* (Vol. 26). New York, NY: Routledge.

Sundberg, J. (1994). Perceptual aspects of singing. *Journal of Voice, 8*, 106–122.

Sundberg, J., & Romedahl, C. (2009). Text intelligibility and the singer's formant—A relationship? *Journal of Voice, 23*(5), 539–545.

Titze, I. (1982). Why is the verbal message less intelligible in singing than in speech? *Journal of Singing, 3*, 37.

Welch, G. F., & Sundberg, J. (2002). "Solo voice." In R. Parncutt & G. E. McPherson (Eds.), *The science and psychology of music performance: Creative strategies for teaching and learning* (pp. 253–268). New York, NY: Oxford University Press.

Index